CRITICAL THINKING IN MEDICAL-SURGICAL SETTINGS
A Case Study Approach

Maryl L. Winningham, APRN, PhD, FACSM
Assistant Professor
and
Barbara A. Preusser, APRN, PhD, CCRN
Assistant Professor

University of Utah College of Nursing
Salt Lake City, Utah 84112

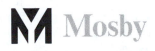 Mosby

St. Louis Baltimore Boston Carlsbad Chicago Naples New York Philadelphia Portland
London Madrid Mexico City Singapore Sydney Tokyo Toronto Wiesbaden

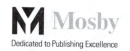

Mosby

Dedicated to Publishing Excellence

A Times Mirror
Company

Publisher: Nancy L. Coon
Editor: Michael S. Ledbetter
Senior Developmental Editor: Teri Merchant
Project Supervisor: Gayle Morris
Cover Design: David Zielinski

Printed in the United States of America

Mosby-Year Book, Inc.
11830 Westline Industrial Drive, St. Louis, Missouri 63146

International Standard Book Number 0-8151-9419-6

96 97 98 99 90 00 / 9 8 7 6 5 4 3 2 1

CONTRIBUTORS

Kathleen Baldwin, RN, PhD, CEN, CCRN
Assistant Professor
College of Nursing
University of Utah
Salt Lake City, Utah
(Multiple system disorders)

Julie Balk, MS, ANP
Advanced Nurse Practitioner
The Heart Center of Salt Lake
Salt Lake City, Utah
(Genitourinary, cardiovascular
disorders)

Nancy Brazelton, RN, MS
Clinical Instructor
College of Nursing
University of Utah
Salt Lake City, Utah
(Neurologic disorders)

Sheryl Davey, RN, MS
Assistant Professor (Clinical)
College of Nursing
University of Utah
Salt Lake City, Utah
(Cardiovascular disorders)

Cynthia Godsey, FNP, MS
Health Care Consultant
Salt Lake City, Utah
(Respiratory disorders)

Carol Green-Nigro, RN, PhD
Nursing Instructor
Johnson County Community College
Overland Park, Kansas
(Immunologic disorders)

Lynn Hollister, RN,C, MS
Nursing Practice Coordinator
HCA St. Marks Hospital
Salt Lake City, Utah
(Introduction to *Instructor's Manual*;
Genitourinary disorders)

Kathleen Kaufman, RN, MS
Assistant Professor (Clinical)
College of Nursing
University of Utah
Salt Lake City, Utah
(Gastrointestinal disorders)

Penny Marshall, RN, PhD
Nursing Instructor
Johnson County Community College
Overland Park, Kansas
(Endocrine disorders)

Shirley Otto, RN, MSN, AOCN, CRNI
Clinical Nurse Specialist
St. Francis Regional Medical Center
Wichita, Kansas
(Hematologic, oncologic disorders)

Barbara A. Preusser, APRN, PhD, CCRN
Assistant Professor
College of Nursing
University of Utah
Salt Lake City, Utah
(Pulmonary, gastrointestinal,
endocrine, and neurological disorders;
emergency situations)

Janet Reilly, RN, MS, CCRN
Assistant Professor (Clinical)
College of Nursing
University of Utah
Salt Lake City, Utah
(Pulmonary disorders)

Janyce Streeter, RN, MS, CCRN
Instructor
College of Nursing
Brigham Young University
Provo, Utah
(Musculoskeletal disorders)

Mary Jo Westin, RN, MS
Instructor
College of Nursing
Brigham Young University
Provo, Utah
(Musculoskeletal disorders)

Russ Wilshaw, RN, MS, CEA
Instructor
College of Nursing
Brigham Young University
Provo, Utah
(Musculoskeletal disorders)

Maryl L. Winningham, APRN, PhD, FACSM
Assistant Professor
College of Nursing
University of Utah
Salt Lake City, Utah
(Instructor's manual; Cardiovascular, endocrine, hematologic, musculoskeletal, and oncologic disorders)

Barbara J. Wirick, RN, MS, CEN
Assistant Professor
Weber State University
Ogden, Utah
(Emergency situations, endocrine disorders)

CONSULTANTS

Kathleen Baldwin, RN, PhD, CEN, CCRN
Assistant Professor
College of Nursing
University of Utah
Salt Lake City, Utah

Brian Barker, RPh
Clinical Pharmacist
Health Science Center
University of Utah
Salt Lake City, Utah
(Pharmacological science)

Sheila A. Dunn, RN, MSN, ANP
Clinical Instructor
St. Louis University
St. Louis, Missouri
Adult Nurse Practitioner
Southern Illiois Healthcare Foundation
Centerville, Illinois

Renata J. M. Engler, MD, COL, MC, USA
Allergy-Immunology Service
Walter Reed Army Medical Center
Washington, DC

L. Joan Goe, RN, EdD
Associate Professor
College of Nursing
University of Utah
Salt Lake City, Utah

Kim Litwack, RN, PhD, CPAN
Associate Professor
College of Nursing
University of New Mexico
Albuquerque, New Mexico

Judith L. Myers, RN, MSN
Assistant Professor
St. Louis University
St. Louis, Missouri

Linda K. Olinger, BS, BSMT, ASCP
Medical Technologist
Summa Health Systems
Akron, Ohio
(Laboratory Science)

Nimmi Welikala-Rasiah, RN, MSN, CCRN
Instructor
University of Nevada-Las Vegas
Las Vegas, Nevada

Linda J. Winningham, RD, MS
Ray, Michigan
(Nutritional Science)

Barbara J. Wirick, RN, MS, CEN
Assistant Professor
Weber State University
Ogden, Utah

To our students,
"who taught us everything we thought we knew!"

M.L.W. & B.A.P

ACKNOWLEDGMENTS

We would like to thank:

- Our patients who let us learn nursing by practicing on them.
- Those nurses we saw in action and told ourselves, "Now *that's* a *great nurse*!"
- The teachers who encouraged us to follow our convictions.

To them we humbly acknowledge our gratitude and indebtedness.

This book would never have become a reality if it weren't for the forbearance and help of the following individuals:

- Sue Meeks, whose job (and talent) it was to organize the raw material and make everything look good.
- Teri Merchant, Senior Development Editor, who tried to keep us on the straight and narrow, patiently listened to us complain, coordinated the review process, and edited this work.
- Michael Ledbetter, Editor, who made this book a reality, and Julie Council, Editorial Assistant, for their support.
- Our consultants and contributors, for the creative work they shared with us.
- Our colleagues and friends who put up with us during the months of heavy writing.
- Our dogs, who felt neglected over the past few months, and who will probably take a copy of this book and bury it deeply in the back yard.

M.L.W. & B.A.P.

INTRODUCTION

Pointers for Students:
How To Look Like You Know What You Are Doing

Clinical experiences can be overwhelming and confusing; the environment is filled with distractions. It doesn't look at all like the book! The following are "tips and tricks" contributed by the writers of these cases. They have been included in the hope that there might be some points you will find useful. Don't read them all at once; read a few here and a few there, and apply them as you get the opportunity.

General Suggestions

- There are five instruments every nursing student should carry at all times. Never lend these items to anyone unless you can afford to replace one or more without complaint. They are a good black ink, ballpoint pen; a good stethoscope; a pocket penlight—preferably with pupil sizes or centimeter ruler on the side; a medium-sized hemostat (straight Kelley); and bandage scissors. Purchase a good quality stethoscope. Try listening with several different types, and choose the one that is best for you—engrave your name on it. The stethoscope is your most important tool.
- Staying hydrated will help you stay more alert. Drink plenty of fluids (besides, it gives you an excuse to go to the bathroom for a 30-second break).
- Keep a quick snack handy. Sometimes you need a pick-me-up and don't have time to leave the unit to get something.
- Plan something special you can do to help alleviate stress, and stick to your plan on a regular basis.
- Use of slang or words that could offend the patients should be avoided. Be aware of your patient's comfort level.
- Assume nothing and take nothing for granted.
- Listen and observe carefully. Be aware of changes and try to anticipate their significance.
- Watch how nurses do things, and pick out things that work best for you.
- Projecting confidence and a "matter of fact" manner will usually put the patient, and yourself, at ease.
- Care should always be taken to respect each patient's privacy; conduct interviews and examinations in a professional manner.
- Be sensitive to hesitation and nonverbal cues when gathering information. What is left unsaid may be extremely important. Use phrases such as "could you tell me more," or "could you help me understand..." to elicit more information.
- Watch for physical or emotional scars. Individuals—both men and women—who have been subjected to the degradation of sexual abuse and molestation may be especially prone to shame, aversion, or aggressive reactions.
- Don't be surprised to find that many adults may not be knowledgeable about the basics of elimination and sexual functioning. This often is covered up by humor.
- Documentation is critical, tools should be simple to use and developed for use at a 6th grade reading level. If you have a limited budget and a clinical setting of patients who speak more than one language, ask for volunteers to help translate educational material.
- As the patient's resting respiratory rate doubles from baseline, s/he will need to be intubated and placed on mechanical ventilation.

- Never trust equipment. Double check to make sure all equipment is functional.
- Treat the patient, not the monitoring devices or numbers.
- Not every patient with hepatitis or cirrhosis is an alcoholic.
- Not every alcoholic will go into DT.
- Do not assume the patient is anorexic if s/he looks malnourished.
- Do not assume a patient is well-nourished just because s/he is obese.

Assessment

Learn to assess pain without leaving out important data. Suggestion: use the COLDERRA method where C = characteristics, O = onset, L = location, D = duration, E = exacerbation, R = relief, R = radiation, and A = associated signs and symptoms.

- Begin with the basics and keep reviewing them: Airway, Breathing, Circulation (ABC).
- Become a keen observer; use all your senses.
- Don't be distracted by the obvious. Keep looking!
- Formulate a systematic way of assessing patients and make it a habit. You will be less likely to overlook or omit something.
- You can't find something if you don't look for it.
- Don't trust (1) machines, (2) numbers, (3) what you can't see.
- With the first assessment of your shift, check the patient's ID bracelet and the rate and type of every fluid infusing — *you* are responsible for fluids under your control from the moment of shift change until your shift is over.
- Remember to auscultate before palpating: Watch! Listen! *Then* Touch!
- Testing pH of NGT drainage is easier if you slip the litmus paper into the end of the NGT and reconnect the tube to suction. Drainage will be pulled over the paper which can then be removed. (Of course, antacids in the tube will negate this.)
- Any abrupt change in color or amount of drainage from drains or wounds needs to be explored and reported.
- Do not suggest words to describe feelings or events to your patients. You may miss subtle nuances if you jump to conclusions; listen to what your patients have to say and how they say it.
- Perform a thorough psychosocial assessment that includes the values of patients and their significant others.
- Include the significant other when you assess sleep patterns. They may be able to tell you more about snoring and other sleep disturbances than the patient can.
- Accurate records of data, such as intake and output, is a must. Lawsuits have been won — and lost — over one single I/O sheet. Involve the patient and family in helping keep records.
- Always double check calculations; use a calculator, if necessary.
- Acute cardiovascular and musculoskeletal injuries require frequent evaluation and documentation of the 5 Ps: Pulse, Pallor, Pain, Paresthesia, and Paralysis. Deterioration of status in any of these variables may indicate a medical emergency.
- Be alert for substance abuse as an underlying diagnosis in individuals whose hospitalization is sudden and unanticipated. Many nurses have been injured by patients in undiagnosed withdrawal. This may be a particular risk in motor vehicle accidents (MVAs) or medical crises, where alcohol or drug use may be contributing factors.

Problem/Diagnoses

- You have gathered your data, now look at it. Do you see any patterns? Do the data fit the history?

- Ask the following questions:
  - Do the data make sense in the context of this patient?
  - Do the data create a complete picture?
  - Do you need additional data?
- Use the data to formulate your list of patient problems.
- Prioritize specific problem statements, and guard yourself against distractions.
- Never be too smart to look something up.

Planning

- Plan and coordinate care with your patient. By discussing interventions and priorities, you will learn to understand more about your patient's value system.
- Noncompliance is rare when there is true teamwork.
- Educate the patient as you carry out this process; process and outcome can and should be integrated. A better educated patient is more prepared to comply with the medical and nursing care regimen.
- Always include relationships, self-esteem, and emotional issues in planning care.
- Prevent infection. Teach your patients and their families to wash their hands properly. Take them to the sink in the room and demonstrate hand washing techniques that you were taught in Nursing 101. Show them how to use a paper towel to turn off the faucet. Have them practice.
- Check equipment; double check if you have any doubt. You are responsible for reporting equipment that is not in working order.
- Substance abuse is not uncommon in the recovery of trauma patients. Consider a psychiatric nurse practitioner or social services consultation if you suspect this is a problem.

Implementation

- Frequently check your patient's charts for STAT orders.
- Document everything you do; if it isn't charted, you didn't do it.
- Document the patient's response to treatments, medications, and activities.
- Let the patient's values and preferences be the guide.
- Get the family and significant others to help, if appropriate.

Evaluation

- Monitor carefully for changes, whether dramatic and sudden, or subtle and gradual.
- Include the patient in helping evaluate care. Ask, "Do you feel that what we have done is helping? What do you think?"
- Is the patient getting better? If yes, then continue with the plan. If not, reassess and revise the plan as needed.
- Evaluate patients' and spousal cooperation. Never label patients as "noncompliant." Determine why patients do not take their medication, complete treatments, etc. The side effects of treatment make him/her feel worse than the disease, and s/he is exercising their right of choice. "Noncompliance" on the part of the patient is more often "knowledge deficit" on our part!
- Long-term problems, particularly pain, often contribute to depression. Involve other health care professionals and pain specialists in addressing these complex issues.

CONTENTS

CHAPTER 1. CARDIOVASCULAR DISORDERS

Case Study 1

Name: _____ *Class/Group:* _____ *Date:* _____

Instructions: All questions apply to this case study. Your response should be brief and to the point. Adequate space has been provided for answers. When asked to provide several answers, they should be listed in order of priority or significance. Do not assume information that is not provided. Please print or write legibly.

You have just accepted a new position as an office RN for a busy internal medicine physician. During your interviews with her, she told you that patient education was very important to her but she has found that she never has enough time to give adequate teaching. Part of your new job is to help her with patient management and education in her already-established hypertension clinic.

On your first day at the hypertension clinic, you meet M.P., a 78 year-old-woman who was told about 6 months ago that her blood pressure was elevated. You take her blood pressure using the 1993 American Heart Association guidelines and get 160/102. She tells you that the physician told her she has hypertension and that she should take a pill everyday. She seems confused and asks you, "What is hypertension, anyway?"

1. How would you explain hypertension to M.P.?

M.P. goes on to say that she feels just fine and doesn't think she needs this pill anyway. She shows you a prescription for enalapril (Vasotec) 2.5 mg daily and states, "The doctor gave this to me but I don't think I'll get it filled. Right now I feel fine."

2. What is your next nursing intervention?

M.P. thanks you for explaining everything to her and reports she will get her prescription filled today on the way home from the doctor's office. She goes on to ask if there is anything else she should do to treat her HTN.

3.   What nonpharmacologic measures might help someone like M.P. control her blood pressure?

M.P. leaves your office a much more informed health care consumer and says she will see you in a month at her follow-up appointment. M.P. returns to the office 4 weeks later. She sits down to get her blood pressure taken and tells you she has been doing everything you taught her and has no questions about your previous teaching.

4.   You are getting ready to take M.P.'s blood pressure. What are important factors to keep in mind to guarantee an accurate reading of M.P.'s blood pressure?

You escort M.P. to the exam room. While you are walking with her she tells you that she has a cough that has been bothering her for the past 3 weeks. She reports it is so bad that she can't even sleep. She tells you she is going to ask the doctor "for an antibiotic to get rid of this cough."

5.   Knowing what you do about M.P.'s treatment plan, what is the most likely cause of her cough?

M.P. sees the physician and tells you that the doctor stopped her medication to see if her cough got better. She has substituted metoprolol (Lopressor) 50 mg bid. M.P. is curious what side effects this new medication will have.

6.   List 4 things you would include in teaching M.P. about her new medication.

M.P. calls you 3 weeks later and states she is feeling fine and does not have any side effects from her new medication. She has had her blood pressure checked twice at the senior citizens' center, and those readings were 138/78 and 142/82.

7.   M.P. asks if these blood pressures readings are OK. What do you tell her?

M.P. comes in for routine follow-up 1 year later. She continues to do well on her metoprolol 50 mg daily with average BP readings of 132/78. She participates in a routine walking program and eats a low-fat, no added salt diet. She tells you she recently was at a luncheon with her garden club and that most of those ladies take different blood pressure pills than she does. She is curious if she would be better off on a different medication.

8.   How can you best respond to M.P.'s statement?

Case Study 2

As an occupational health nurse at a free-standing HMO clinic, one of your primary responsibilities is providing information to all employees on healthy lifestyles. While you are waiting in the supermarket check-out line, your neighbors seek you out for advice. He reports that he recently had a physical and was given a "clean bill of health." He tells you he feels great but confides in you that his family history of premature coronary disease worries him. He said he wants to limit his risk factors but he just doesn't know what to do. You agree to see him later in the week to guide him in identifying lifestyle changes he can make.

During your initial interview you learn that K.N. is 55 years old and has no chronic medical problems. His family history is significant for premature coronary artery disease in both his father and mother. His father experienced his first MI at the age of 49 and his mother died of an MI at the age of 60. He has never smoked and denies any hypertension, diabetes, or other medical problems. He is 5'10" and weighs 200 lb. His VS are 128/70, 72, 16. He has a sedentary job and gets no routine exercise. He gives you a lipid profile laboratory analysis that reveals the following values: total cholesterol 243 mg/dl, LDL 165 mg/dl, HDL 31 mg/dl, triglycerides 240 mg/dl.

1. His waist and hip circumferences are 48.5" and 40.5", respectively. Describe at what location and how these measurements are made.

2. Calculate K.N.'s WHR, and explain the significance of your finding.

3. Identify all the cardiac-related risk factors in K.N.'s previous information. Place a check mark (✓) next to those that are modifiable risk factors

4.   Based on the information you received in the initial interview, what lifestyle modifications would you prescribe for K.N.?

You and K.N. decide that his first efforts will be directed toward dietary modification. Successful dietary modification could help his weight loss efforts, as well as his hyperlipidemia.

5.   What information would you give to K.N. regarding a healthy diet?

The 1993 National Cholesterol Education Program (NCEP) recommendation for initial diet therapy is called a Step 1 Diet. This involves reduction of dietary fat to less than 30% of total calories and a reduction of saturated fat to less than 10% of total calories. Cholesterol intake is limited to less than 300 mg/day. More recent data suggest that a very low-fat diet (less than 20% fat) may be more effective where CAD already exists.

K.N. already appears overwhelmed and states, "Just tell me how I can do this in my everyday life."

6.   How would you explain this to him in plain English?

K.N. tells you he was not fasting when his lipid profile was drawn. He is curious if this made his cholesterol higher than it really is.

7.   How would you answer K.N.'s question?

You write down the name of two inexpensive books on low-fat, healthy eating that K.N. can get locally. K.N. sets up a follow-up appointment with you in 2 months. When he returns, he has the results of his most recent lipid profile. The results are total cholesterol 220 mg/dl, LDL 143 mg/dl, HDL 32 mg/dl, and triglycerides 165 mg/dl. His vital signs remain within normal limits. He has lost 8 lb since you last saw him; even better, his WHR is 1.12!

8.   What diet instruction would you give K.N. now?

K.N. states he understands the goal for his LDL cholesterol is less than 190 and that LDL is his "bad" cholesterol. He questions what his goal is for his HDL cholesterol and is curious if this is what people mean by "good" cholesterol.

9.   What information would you give K.N. about HDL cholesterol?

K.N. verbalizes understanding of the teaching regarding HDL cholesterol. He feels he adequately understands his diet therapy and would now like to start a routine exercise program.

10. What general information would you give him regarding an exercise program?

K.N. follows up with you in 2 months. He has lost an additional 10 pounds and feels great. More important, his WHR is 0.93. He denies any problems regarding his dietary or exercise programs and expresses appreciation for your help. His repeat HDL is 50 mg/dl and LDL is 130 mg/dl.

Case Study 3

Name: _____ Class/Group: _____ Date: _____

Instructions: All questions apply to this case study. Your response should be brief and to the point. Adequate space has been provided for answers. When asked to provide several answers, they should be listed in order of priority or significance. Do not assume information that is not provided. Please print or write legibly.

You are a nurse at a free-standing cardiac prevention and rehabilitation center. Your new client in risk-factor modification is B.J., a 37-year-old traveling salesman, who is married with 3 children. During a recent evaluation for chest pain (including a cardiac catheterization), he was diagnosed with angina pectoris, given a prescription for SL nitroglycerin, told how to use it, and referred to your cardiac rehabilitation program for sessions 3 days a week. B.J.'s wife comes along to help him with healthy lifestyle changes. You take the following nursing history: B.J.'s father died of sudden cardiac death at age 42 and his mother (still living) had a CABG x 4 (quadruple coronary artery bypass graft of 4 vessels) at age 52; his hypertension is controlled with nifedipine (Procardia) 90 mg PO qd, which he has taken regularly; he has a 35 pack/year smoking history; an occasional beer ("a beer every weekend with the football game"); and a dietary history of fried and fast foods. His current weight is 205 at 5'8"; waist/hip ratio of 1.21. His VS are 132/86, 82, 18, 98.4°F.

1. List 3 nonmodifiable risk factors for CAD.

2. List 6 modifiable risk factors for CAD.

3. Underline each of the responses in #1 and #2 above that represent B.J.'s CAD risk factors.

4. You would like to know more about B.J.'s hyperlipidemia. What 4 common laboratory values do you need to know?

B.J. laughingly tells you he believes in the 5 all-American food groups: salt, sugar, fat, chocolate and caffeine.

5. Identify health-related problems in this case description; the problem that is potentially life-threatening should be listed first.

6. What is the most important priority problem that you need to address with B.J.? Identify the teaching strategy you would use with him.

7. What is the second problem you would work with B.J. to change? Identify an appropriate strategy to resolve the problem.

8. B.J.'s wife takes you aside and tells you, "I'm so worried for B. I grew up in a really dysfunctional family where there was a lot of violence. B. has been so good to the kids and me. I'm so worried I'll lose him that I have nightmares about his heart stopping. I find myself suddenly awakening at night just to see if he's breathing." How are you going to respond?

Note: Nightmares about losing a loved one to heart disease are not rare, especially during the time of diagnosis or disease-related crisis. However, a background of childhood violence can have deep roots and often requires special help. Clearly, this is woman is in distress. Depending on her willingness at this time, it would be good for her to talk with a therapist. If she doesn't think she needs it, try suggesting that it might be good for B. and the kids and that it would help her relax and be more responsive to them. At the appropriate point, it would be important for her to be able to share with B. how she feels. From her description, this sleep disturbance is an unhealthy situation that should be addressed. If she refuses, keep an open relationship; it is important that she keep talking to someone about her fear.

9. Six weeks after you start working with B.J., he admits that he has been under a lot of stress. He rubs his chest and says, "It feels really heavy on my chest right now." You feel his pulse and note that his skin is slightly diaphoretic, he is agitated, and appears to be very anxious. What are you going to do to obtain additional information?

10. B.J. continues to feel symptomatic. Now what are you going to do?

Case Study 4

W.R., a 48-year-old construction worker with a 36-pack/year smoking history, is admitted to your floor with a diagnosis of rule out myocardial infarction (R/O MI). He has significant male-pattern obesity ("beer belly," high WHR), a barrel chest, and reports a dietary history of high-fat food. His wife brought him to the ED after he complained of unrelieved "indigestion." His admission VS were 202/124, 96, 18, 36.8°C. W.R. was put on O_2 2 L/nc, an IV of D_5W at KVO was started, and he was given sublingual nifedipine (Procardia) in the ED. He was admitted to Dr. Adam's service. He tells you he's just fine in a loud and angry voice and demands a cigarette.

1. Are these VS reasonable for a man his age? If not, which one(s) concern(s) you. State your reasons why?

2. Identify 5 priority problems associated with the care of a patient like W.R.

3. List 3 relevant nursing diagnoses for a cardiac patient like W.R.

4. Which of the following laboratory tests might be ordered to investigate W.R.'s condition? If the order is appropriate, place an "A" in the space provided.
    ___ CBC.
    ___ EEG in the AM.
    ___ Chem 7 (electrolytes).
    ___ PT/PTT.
    ___ Bilirubin q AM.
    ___ Urinalysis.
    ___ STAT 12-lead ECG.
    ___ Type and cross (T & C) for 4 units PRCs (packed red cells)

5. What significant laboratory tests are missing from the above list?

6. How are you going to respond to his angry demands for a cigarette? He also demands something for his "heartburn." How will you respond?

You call Dr. Adam's resident who prescribes 10 mg morphine sulphate IV push q1h prn for pain (burning, pressure, angina).

7. Explain 2 reasons for this order.

8. What special precautions should you follow when administering morphine sulfate IV push?

9. What safety measures/instructions would you give him before you leave his room?

10. One of the housekeeping staff asks you, "If the poor guy can't smoke, why can't you give him a nicotine patch?" How will you respond?

11. Before leaving for the night, Mrs. R. approaches you and asks, "Did W. have a heart attack? I'm really scared. His father died of one when he was 51." How are you going to respond to her question?

12. When you come into W.R.'s at 2200 to answer his call light, you see he is holding his left arm and complaining of aching in his left shoulder and arm? What information are you going to gather? What questions will you ask him?

13. Based on your assessment findings, you decide to call the physician. What information are you going to report to her?

It was determined that W. R. has coronary artery disease (CAD). The physician suggested it would be best to treat him medically for now. He was discharged with a referral for a follow-up visit to the cardiologist in 1 week.

14. Before discharge, what 4 educational issues are you going to discuss with W.R. and his wife?

Case Study 5

You are assigned to care for L.J., a 70-year-old retired bus driver who has just been admitted to your medical floor with R leg deep vein thrombosis (DVT). L.J. has a 48 pack/year smoking history, although he states he quit 2 years ago. He has had pneumonia several times, frequent episodes of atrial fibrillation, 2 previous episodes of DVT, and was diagnosed with rheumatoid arthritis 3 years ago. Two months ago he began experiencing shortness of breath on exertion and noticed swelling of his R foreleg that became progressively worse until it also involved his thigh to the groin. His wife brought him to the hospital when he complained of increasingly severe pain in his leg. When a Doppler study indicated a probable thrombus of the external iliac vein extending distally to the lower leg, he was admitted for bed rest and IV heparin therapy. Significant admission lab values are: PT 12.4 sec, PTT 25 sec, Hgb 13.3 g/dl, Hct 38.9% mg/dl, cholesterol 206 mg/dl. Electrolytes are normal.

1. List 6 risk factors for DVT.

2. Identify the problems from L.J.'s history above that represent his personal risk factors.

3. Keeping in mind L. J.'s health history and admitting diagnosis, what are the most important assessments you should make during your physical examination and assessment?

4. What is the most serious complication of DVT?

Your assessment of L.J. reveals bibasilar crackles with moist cough; normal heart sounds, BP 138/88, P 104, 3+ pitting edema R lower extremity, mild erythema of R foot and calf, and severe R calf pain. He is alert and oriented but a little restless. He denies shortness of breath and chest pain.

5.   Which of these assessment findings should you monitor closely for development of the complication identified in #4?

6.   List 6 other common signs/symptoms of this complication in order of priority.

Note: If a pulmonary embolism is massive, the signs/symptoms are more like those of myocardial infarction: crushing, substernal chest pain, marked respiratory distress, feeling of impending doom, rapid, shallow breathing, dysrhythmias, shock.

You place L.J. on bed rest and give him a bolus of 5000 units of heparin SC, followed by a continuous IV heparin drip. You give him acetaminophen (Tylenol) as ordered, for pain.

7.   The heparin comes premixed as heparin 20,000 units in 500 ml D_5W. If the physician prescribed the patient to receive 1240 U/h, how fast would you infuse the drip? What will be the method of infusion?

8.   What instructions will you give him about his activity?

Note: Significant others often want to do something helpful. Having them remind the patient to do their ankle exercises, in particular, can be a valuable adjunct.

9.   What pertinent laboratory values/test results would you expect the physician to order (and that you should monitor)?

10. One of your nursing diagnoses/patient problems is pain. List 4 interventions you would choose for L.J. associated with this diagnosis?

A week has passed. L.J. responded to heparin therapy, was started on warfarin (Coumadin) therapy, and is being discharged to home for home care follow-up. "Good," he says, "just in time to fly out West for my grandson's wedding." His wife, who has come to pick him up, rolls her eyes and looks at the ceiling. You almost drop the discharge papers in disbelief at what you have just heard (and you thought you did such a good job of discharge teaching!).

11. What are you going to say to him?

L.J. listened to you and Mrs. J. was quite relieved (she has been telling her friends about this "wonderful nurse who talked some sense into my husband"). L.J.'s son arranged to video-tape the entire ceremony and guests at the reception taped special greetings for him. It's been 2 weeks and he seems quite pleased. He watches the tape daily and points out his favorite parts to the home care nurse every time she visits.

Case Study 6

Name: _____ *Class/Group:* _____ *Date:* _____

Instructions: All questions apply to this case study. Your response should be brief and to the point. Adequate space has been provided for answers. When asked to provide several answers, they should be listed in order of priority or significance. Do not assume information that is not provided. Please print or write legibly.

You are just getting caught up with your work when you receive the following phone call, "Hi, this is Deb in the ED. We're sending you M.M., a 63-year-old Hispanic woman with a PMH of CAD. Her daughter reports that she's become increasingly weaker over the last couple weeks and has been unable to do her housework. Apparently she has been c/o swelling in her ankles and feet by late afternoon, and has nocturnal diuresis x 4. Her daughter brought her in because she has complained of heaviness in her chest off and on over the last few days but denies any discomfort at this time. The daughter, N., took her to see her family physician who immediately sent her here. VS are 146/92, 96, 24, 37.2°C. She has an IV of D_5W at KVO in her right forearm. Her labs are as follows: Na 134 mEq/L, K 3.5 mEq/L, Cl 103 mEq/L, HCO_3 23, BUN 13 mg/dl, creatinine 1.3 mg/dl, glucose 153 mg/dl, WBC 8.3 mm³, Hct 33.9%, Hgb 11.7 g/dl, platelets 162 mm³. PT, PTT, and UA are pending. She has had her CXR and ECG and her orders have been written."

1. What additional information do you need from the ED nurse?

2. How are you going to prepare for this patient?

3. M. M. arrives by wheelchair (w/c). As she transfers from the w/c to the bed, what observations should you make?

4. Given the information above, which of the following orders would be appropriate for this patient? Carefully review each order to determine if it is appropriate or inappropriate as written. If the order is appropriate, place an "A" in the space provided; if the order is inappropriate, place an "I" in the space provided and underline the inappropriate part.
   ___ Routine VS.
   ___ Serum magnesium STAT.
   ___ Up ad lib.
   ___ 10 g sodium, low animal fat diet.
   ___ Change IV to NS at 100 ml/h.
   ___ Cardiac enzymes on admission and q8h x 24 then q AM.
   ___ CBC, Chem 7 and lipid profile in AM.
   ___ Schedule for abdominal CT scan for AM.
   ___ Heparin 10,000 U sq q8h.
   ___ Docusate sodium 100 mg PO, qd.
   ___ Ampicillin 250 mg IVPB q6h.
   ___ Furosemide 200 mg IVP STAT.
   ___ Nitroglycerin 0.4 mg 1 SL q4h prn for chest pain.

5. When you respond to M.M.'s call light, you observe she is talking rapidly in Spanish and pointing to the bathroom. Her speech pattern indicates she is SOB. You assist her to the bathroom and note that her skin feels clammy. While sitting on the commode she vomits. On a scale of 1 to 10 (1 = being no problem, 10 = being a CODE-level emergency), how would you rate this situation and why?

6. Identify at least 4 actions you should take next, and state your rationale.

Note: If a physician is not immediately available and/or the staffing is such that you can not obtain adequate help, do not hesitate to call a CODE. This is an urgent situation.

7. The physician calls your unit to find out what is happening. What information would you need to convey at this time?

8. The resident is coming to the floor to evaluate the patient immediately. In the meantime she orders Lasix 40 mg IVP STAT. You only have 20 mg in stock. Should you give the 20 mg now, then give the additional 20 mg when it comes up from pharmacy?

9. M.M. continues to experience vomiting and diaphoresis that are unrelieved by medication and comfort measures. A STAT 12-lead ECG reveals ischemic changes. The patient is transferred to the coronary care unit. As you give report to the receiving RN, what laboratory value is the most important to report and why?

10. While recovering in ICU, M.M. slipped in the bathroom and fractured her femur. Because of the surgical risks involved, M. M. was treated conservatively and put in a long leg cast. She is again transferred to your floor. A geriatric nurse practitioner (GNP) has been asked to evaluate M.M.'s home to see if she can be discharged to her own home or will need to stay elsewhere. Identify 8 things that the GNP would assess.

11. Since it was determined that M.M. lived in an apartment with poor access, she elected to stay with her daughter and 5 grandchildren in their small home. A home care nurse comes 3 times a week to check on her. M.M. is easily fatigued and the children are quite lively. Suggest some ways the daughter can ensure that her mother isn't overwhelmed and doesn't become exhausted in this situation.

Case Study 7

Name: _____ *Class/Group:* _____ *Date:* _____

Instructions: All questions apply to this case study. Your response should be brief and to the point. Adequate space has been provided for answers. When asked to provide several answers, they should be listed in order of priority or significance. Do not assume information that is not provided. Please print or write legibly.

R.K. is a 90-year-old woman who lives with her husband of the same age. Two nights before her admission to your cardiac floor, she awoke with heavy, substernal pressure accompanied by epigastric distress. The pain was reduced somewhat when she rolled onto her side but did not completely subside for about 6 hours. The next night she experienced the same chest pressure. The following morning, R.K.'s husband took her to the doctor and she was subsequently hospitalized to rule out myocardial infarction (R/O MI).

You obtain the following information from your nursing history and physical exam: R.K. has no history of smoking or alcohol use; has been in good general health with the exception of osteoarthritis of her hands and knees and some osteoporosis of the spine; and her only medications are ranitidine (Zantac), ibuprofen (Motrin) for bone and joint pain, and "herbs." On admission her VS are 142/84, 88, 16, 37.2°C; weight 52 kg. Trace edema of both ankles is present, but capillary refill and peripheral pulses are 1 +. You hear a soft systolic murmur. You place her on telemetry, which shows frequent PACs but no ventricular ectopy. She is not in any discomfort at present.

1. R. K. became fatigued during the admission process and you decide to let her sleep. When she wakes, what additional history and physical information should you obtain related to her admitting diagnosis?
   History

   Physical Exam

2. List 7 lab/diagnostic tests that you would expect the physician to order, and suggest what each may contribute.

3. What other source, besides cardiac, might be responsible for her chest and abdominal discomfort (specify)?

4. Differentiate between pain of ischemic cardiac origin and that of noncardiac origin.

5. Define the concept "differential diagnosis" and explain what it means.

6. Explain how the concept of differential diagnosis applies to R.K.'s symptoms?

7. Florence Nightingale frequently emphasized the value of good observation skills in nurses. Explain how a good nursing assessment can contribute to making the differential diagnosis.

8. Abnormalities on R.K.'s 12-lead ECG were reported as "slight left axis deviation." Serial CPKs are: 27 U/ml, 24 U/ml, 26 U/ml; first LDH is 215 U/ml. A series of tests ruled out a noncardiac cause for her chest pain. On the basis of the information presented so far, do you believe that she has had a myocardial infarction? What is your rationale?

9. While you care for R.K. you carefully monitor her. Identify 2 possible complication of CAD and the signs/symptoms associated with each.

10. R.K. rings her call bell. When you arrive, she places her hand over her heart and tells you she is "having that terrible heavy feeling again." She is not diaphoretic or nauseated but states she is short of breath. What can you do to make her more comfortable?

Note: CPK can be reported in terms of U/ml or U/L. Always read laboratory reports carefully to be sure which units are used in your institution.

Case Study 8

C.C., a 60-year-old single, retired real estate agent, has a long history of cardiovascular disease due to generalized atherosclerosis. He also has hypertension and COPD (with home O_2). Three serious MIs in the past resulted in ischemic cardiomyopathy, necessitating a cardiac transplant 9 years ago. He developed chronic renal failure as a result of the cyclosporine he is taking to prevent rejection. Two years ago he had an axillary-bifemoral graft for peripheral vascular occlusion and ultimately required transmetatarsal amputation of the L foot. Three days ago C.C. had an acute onset of R calf pain with numbness, pain, loss of movement, and coldness of the R lower leg and foot. A vascular scan showed complete occlusion of the R side of the axillary-bifemoral graft, and he was admitted to your SICU in preparation for a R above-knee amputation.

His routine medications include azathioprene (Imuran), furozemide (Lasix), cyclosporine (Sandimmune), prednisone, metholazone (Zaroxolyn), hydrocodone with acetaminophen (Vicodin), Lisinopril (Zestril), warfarin (Coumadin), digoxin (Lanoxin), diazepam (Valium), MgOxide, and KCl. Before the surgery, his VS are 140/72, 115, and 20. Significant abnormal lab values are: K 6.0 mEq/L, BUN 150 mg/dl, creatinine 11.2 mg/dl, PT 42.1 sec, PTT 50 sec, WBCs 16.2 mm³, cholesterol 295 mg/dl. Chest x-ray shows clear lungs and cardiomegaly. You hear an S_3 gallop and tricuspid regurgitation murmur on cardiac auscultation. His right leg is without pulses by Doppler from the knee down.

1. What critical history information would you need about C.C. to prepare his discharge planning?

2. What abnormal lab value is of concern, and what would you expect the physician to order to correct it?

3. From the above information, what is the reason for the elevated BUN and creatinine?

4. From the PT and PTT, what complication might you expect after surgery and why?

5.   C. C. will return to the SICU after his surgery, as he has after his previous surgeries. He is very apprehensive about the experience. What can you do to allay his fears?

In the SICU on the third postop day, C.C.'s VS are 122/66, 113, 12. His hemodynamic values are: PCWP 15 mm Hg, central venous pressure (CVP) 11 mm Hg, pulmonary artery pressure (PAP) 28/20 mm Hg, cardiac output 4.5 L/min.

6.   From these values, would you describe his condition as hemodynamically stable?

7.   Large amounts of $D_5\frac{1}{2}$ NS are given to keep rhabdomyolysis from elevating the BUN. What serious complications might the IV fluid cause, and how would you monitor for that complication?

8.   Which medications and electrolytes would you expect to be monitor closely and why?

9.   C.C.'s glucose level is 216 mg/dl on the third postop day. It had been 107 mg/dl the day before surgery. How do you account for this elevation?

10.   C.C. tells you he knows he's being silly, but he's experiencing "terrible sharp pain" in his R lower leg. What are you going to do and why?

Case Study 9

Name: _____ Class/Group: _____ Date: _____

Instructions: All questions apply to this case study. Your response should be brief and to the point. Adequate space has been provided for answers. When asked to provide several answers, they should be listed in order of priority or significance. Do not assume information that is not provided. Please print or write legibly.

J.T. is a 58-year-old Tongan man admitted to your floor with syncope and right-sided heart failure. He was brought to the hospital after "passing out" and "turning blue" for 2 minutes after a severe bout of coughing. Because J.T. speaks very little English, his wife helps you obtain his health history: NIDDM, significant abdominal obesity, hypertension, CHF, chronic hypoxia, frequent pneumonia, hyperlipidemia, and polycythemia. His wife tells you he snores loudly and seems to stop breathing sometimes during the night. He has no history of smoking or alcohol use. His weight is 310 pounds. Over the last week he has had intermittent chest pain with shortness of breath on exertion. The shortness of breath has increased during the last 12 hours. He has been hospitalized in the past for chest pain but has never had an MI. On admission today he has orthopnea, a severe dry cough, palpitations, and shortness of breath. He is not complaining of chest pain or discomfort. His VS are 146/94, 64, 20, 36.7°C. You hear muffled S_1 and S_2 heart sounds and a possible S_3. He has moderate pretibial edema to his knees and a few bibasilar crackles. You place him on oxygen at 3 L/min by nasal cannula and insert a Foley catheter. His blood glucose level is 147 mg/dl and Hct is 50%. Other lab values are normal, including cholesterol and triglyceride levels.

1. What is the relationship of J.T.'s country of origin to his current health problems?

2. What do you think is the significance of J.T.'s wife's report about his snoring and sleep-related breathing pattern?

3. Judging from the admission information, do you think he has right-sided CHF, left-sided CHF, or both? Cite your evidence.

4. List 3 other things you could assess to confirm your suspicion of right-sided failure.

5.   What is a possible explanation for his chronic hypoxia?

6.   List 4 priority nursing diagnoses for J. T.

The night shift nurse confirms the report that J.T. snores loudly ("I could hear him all the way down the hall!") and has 30- to 60-second pauses in his breathing followed by a violent jerk and thrashing as he resumes inspirations. A sleep study is ordered.

7.   Define a sleep study and what information can be obtained from it.

The sleep study showed obstructive sleep apnea with oxygen desaturation as low as 32% for prolonged periods following each apneic episode. During his study, J.T. had over 320 apneic episodes in 1 night.

8.   Continuous positive airway pressure (CPAP) is prescribed for J.T. Explain the concept of CPAP and how it will benefit him.

On the forth day after admission, J.T. developed chills and fever with a temperature of 38.5°C and an SaO_2 of 88% on 3 L O_2/nc.

9.   What are the 2 most likely sources of infection that might be responsible for his fever?

J. T. was diagnosed with pneumonia and started on erythromycin. During his hospitalization, J.T.'s family has repeatedly brought him food and drinks from home in spite of explanations by the nurses that he is on a 2000-calorie, low-salt, diabetic diet, and on fluid restriction. Because of his obesity and extreme shortness of breath on exertion, he is quite immobilized.

10. Identify the most serious complication of immobility for which he is at risk, and state the reasons for this risk.

After a week on erythromycin for his pneumonia and diuresis for his CHF, J.T.'s doctor says he is ready to go home. You have developed a list of things that you think he and his family should be taught before he is ready for discharge. After reviewing his history, you have decided that he has many risk factors for coronary artery disease; although he has not had an MI yet, he is at risk for having one. You have placed teaching about cardiac risk factors at the top of your list.

11. List 4 cardiac risk factors that J. T. has and place a check (✓) mark beside the ones that are potentially modifiable through behavioral change.

Note: Although polycythemia is uncommon and is not on the list of usual coronary risk factors, it increases the tendency for clot formation and increases the risk for MI.

12. Identify 2 major pathologic conditions J.T. has for which he needs teaching.

13. What do you think is the likelihood J.T. will be motivated to exercise and diet to lose weight and why?

Case Study 10

Three years ago, M.Y., a 50-year-old building contractor from Montana, consulted his physician for shortness of breath, fatigue, swelling of his legs, and syncopal episodes. An echocardiogram done at the time revealed an ejection fraction of 25% to 30% with mild mitral regurgitation. M.Y. refused a cardiac catheterization and other invasive tests and procedures, instead choosing to be treated for his CHF with medications (furosemide [Lasix], enalapril [Vasotec] and aspirin). He did well until 3 to 4 months ago when he developed increasing pedal edema, generalized fluid retention, dramatic decrease in activity level, severe dyspnea, and cough. Another echocardiogram showed his ejection fraction had decreased to 12% and that he also had 4-chamber dilation. He was diagnosed with idiopathic dilated cardiomyopathy, hospitalized, and started on dobutamine (Dobutrex) and lidocaine drips. His PCWP was 26 mm Hg and cardiac index 1.8. He was transferred by plane to a large regional medical center because of the seriousness of his condition to await a heart transplant.

M.Y. lives alone. His only living family members are a brother and a sister who both reside in distant states. M.Y. spent 2 weeks in the MICU while his cardiac output and blood pressure were supported by dopamine (Intropin) and dobutamine. The transplant surgery was successful, and he is now recovering on the telemetry unit.

1. You talk with M.Y. about his presurgery experience. Name at least 6 changes in everyday functioning you would you expect a person with advanced CHF to experience.

2. Name at least 5 emotional issues you might expect in an individual with advanced CHF and explain your rationale.

3. Formulate a question to help M.Y. talk about his present feelings.

The transplant team prepares M.Y. for discharge. The social worker is checking into the financial aspects of care in M.Y.'s home community. As the transplant nurse, you have been asked to talk with him about issues relating to his discharge readiness. You decide to start with a psychosocial evaluation to determine problem areas, identify strengths, and determine need for further evaluation and treatment.

4.   What are some potential problem areas related to M.Y.'s transplant you will want to investigate?

5.   What can you do to help him if he has problems in any of the above psychosocial areas?

6.   In order to plan his discharge teaching, you evaluate his understanding of the physical implications of his transplant surgery and the treatments required. List 6 important areas of knowledge you will investigate.

You discover that he understands the anatomy and physiology, record keeping and clinic visits, and medications well after extensive teaching by his physician. However, he has many questions about rejection, infection, activity, and diet. You address these latter issues.

7.   During the first 3 to 6 months after a transplant, most patients experience an episode during which their body tries to reject the new heart. You teach M.Y. that he must contact his physician if he experiences any signs and symptoms of rejection. List 4 signs and symptoms.

8.   List 5 guidelines he should know to guard against infections.

9.   What should M.Y. be taught about diet?

10. M.Y. will begin a regular exercise program shortly after surgery. What should he be taught about activity?

Case Study 11

Name: _____ Class/Group: _____ Date: _____

Instructions: All questions apply to this case study. Your response should be brief and to the point. Adequate space has been provided for answers. When asked to provide several answers, they should be listed in order of priority or significance. Do not assume information that is not provided. Please print or write legibly.

J.F. is a 50-year-old married homemaker with a genetic autoimmune deficiency who has suffered from recurrent bacterial endocarditis. The most recent episodes were a *Staphylococcus aureus* infection of the mitral valve 16 months ago and a *Streptococcus mutans* infection of the aortic valve 1 month ago. During this latter hospitalization, an echocardiogram showed aortic stenosis, moderate aortic insufficiency, chronic valvular vegetations, and moderate atrial enlargement. Two years ago she received an 18-month course of TPN therapy for malnutrition caused by idiopathic, relentless nausea and vomiting. She has also had CAD for several years, and 2 years ago suffered an acute anterior wall MI. In addition, she has a history of chronic joint pain.

Now, after being home for only a week, J.F. has been readmitted to your floor with endocarditis, nausea and vomiting, and renal failure. Since yesterday she has been vomiting and retching constantly, and has had chills, fever, fatigue, joint pain, and headache. As you admit her, you note that she wears glasses and has dentures. She was immediately started on TPN at 125 ml/h and on penicillin 2 million units IV q4h, to be continued for 4 weeks. Other medications are Lasix 80 mg PO qd, amiodipine (Norvasc) 5 mg PO qd, metoprolol 25 mg bid, and droperidol (Inapsine) 0.25-0.5 ml IVP prn for N/V. Admission VS 172/48 (supine) and 100/40 (sitting), 116, 20, 37.9°C. As you assess her, you find a grade II/VI holosystolic murmur and a grade III/VI diastolic murmur; 2+ pitting tibial edema but no peripheral cyanosis; clear lungs; orientation x 3 but drowsiness; soft abdomen with slight tenderness in the L upper quadrant; hematuria; and multiple petechiae on skin of arms, legs, and chest.

1. What is the significance of the orthostatic hypotension, the wide pulse pressure, and the tachycardia?

2. What is the significance of the abdominal tenderness, hematuria, joint pain, and petechiae?

3. As you monitor your patient throughout the day, what other signs and symptoms of embolization will you watch for?

4.   Three important diagnostic criteria for infectious endocarditis are anemia, fever, and cardiac murmurs. Explain the cause for each sign.

5.   On the day after admission, you review J.F.s laboratory test results: Na 138 mEq/L, K 3.9 mEq/L, Cl 103 mEq/L, BUN 85 mg/dl, creatinine 3.9 mg/dl, glucose 185 mg/dl, WBCs 6.7 mm^3, Hct 27%, Hgb 9.0 g/dl. Identify the values that are not within normal ranges, and explain the reason for each abnormality.

6.   What is the greatest risk for J.F. during the process of rehydration and what would you monitor to detect its development?

As you admitted J.F., you were aware that as soon as she is stable, she will be going home in a few days on TPN and IV antibiotics. Therefore, you plan to initiate discharge preparations and teaching as soon as possible.

7.   List 5 questions you might ask in assessing her home health care needs.

Fortunately, J.F. has a supportive husband and 2 daughters who live nearby who can function as caregivers when J.F. is discharged. They, as well as the patient, will also need teaching about endocarditis. Although J.F. has been ill for several years, you discover that she and her family have received little education about the disease. You prepare a teaching plan for the family.

8.   List 2 predisposing causes of bacteremia that you will explain.

9.   List 3 other things you would teach.

10. Your hospital discharge planner facilitates J.F.'s transition to home care. During
     the initial home visit, the home health nurse evaluates J.F.'s IV site for
     implementation of the IV therapy program, and interviews the family members to
     determine their willingness to be caregivers and their level of understanding, and
     enlists the patient's and family's assistance to identify 10 teaching goals. What
     topics would be included on this list?

11. The home health nurse also writes short- and long-term goals for J.F. and her
     family. Identify 2 short- and 3 long-term goals.
     <u>Short-term</u>

     <u>Long term</u>

Mr. F. and his 2 daughters learned to administer her TPN during the 18-month treatment.
Be aware that IV cases are usually covered by most insurers on a case-by-case basis and
with clear documentation.

12. What documentation would be required in order to obtain reimbursement?

Case Study 12

Name: _____ Class/Group: _____ Date: _____

Instructions: All questions apply to this case study. Your response should be brief and to the point. Adequate space has been provided for answers. When asked to provide several answers, they should be listed in order of priority or significance. Do not assume information that is not provided. Please print or write legibly.

L.M. is a 60-year-old woman who is admitted to your telemetry unit in a major medical center after being successfully resuscitated by medics from a cardiac arrest due to ventricular fibrillation. L.M., a divorced housewife, had her sudden death experience in the small rural community where she lives and was transported to your facility for evaluation and treatment after she was stabilized. At the time of her arrest her K level was 2.8 mEq/L and Mg level was low. As you continue to review her medical history, you learn that she had rheumatic fever as a child and over the years has developed severe rheumatic heart disease with mitral and aortic valve involvement and dilated cardiomyopathy. Four years ago she had a commissurotomy for mitral valve prolapse. She also has probable aortic valve stenosis. During the past year she has experienced increasing problems with chest pain, shortness of breath, and dyspnea on exertion. Two months ago she developed a severe cough and increasing fatigue. She has been on furosemide (Lasix) 40 mg PO qd, digoxin (Lanoxin) 0.25 mg PO qd, captopril 50 mg PO q8h, potassium (K Dur) 20 mEq qd, and warfarin (Coumadin) 5 mg PO qd. In addition, during the week before her cardiac arrest, she was taking erythromycin 500 mg q6h for a lower respiratory tract infection. Although she stopped smoking 4 years ago, she had a 40 pack/year smoking history.

1.   What organism causes rheumatic fever?

2.   What medication is commonly used prophylactically to prevent development of rheumatic heart disease when an individual has rheumatic fever?

3.   Why would someone like L.M. be given Coumadin?

4.   Reviewing the above health history, what factors do you think contribute to her current symptoms of chest pain, shortness of breath, dyspnea on exertion, cough, and fatigue? Explain your rationale for each.

5.   What factors in the above health history may have precipitated L.M.'s cardiac arrest?

L.M.'s admission VS are 102/60, 84, 16, and 36°C. Her telemetry monitor shows atrial fibrillation and frequent PVCs. When you listen to her heart, you hear an S_3 gallop, a grade III/VI systolic murmur, and a soft, blowing diastolic murmur. Her PMI is displaced laterally. She has no pedal edema. You hear crackles in her lungs. Other assessment findings are normal. She is transferred to the coronary care unit and is placed on continuous heparin and lidocaine IV infusions, and started on O_2 at 40% by face mask. Her lab values are drawn. Later in the day during a cardiac catheterization, her cardiac output was found to be 2.3 L/min and her mean pulmonary artery pressure 29 mm Hg.

6.   Based on the above assessment, do you believe that L.M. is experiencing some heart failure? Why or why not?

7.   L.M.'s lab tests return. Her PT is 23.4 seconds, PTT 30 seconds. What other lab tests would you especially want to monitor?

8.   Why is it important to monitor L.M.'s PTT? Is her PTT within the therapeutic range? Is the PT within the normal range?

9.   List 4 relevant nursing diagnoses for L.M.

10. In order to prevent serious complications, you will assess and monitor for potential problems. List 3 significant potential physiologic problems for which L.M. is at risk. Explain.

11. The technologic monitoring and care L.M. receives demands so much time that there has been little opportunity to talk with her about her feelings related to her sudden death experience. As you plan to approach her, you remind yourself to be sensitive to communication limitations imposed by her pathologic condition. What are 2 of these, and how will they affect your interaction?

Case Study 13

Name: _____ Class/Group: _____ Date: _____

Instructions: All questions apply to this case study. Your response should be brief and to the point. Adequate space has been provided for answers. When asked to provide several answers, they should be listed in order of priority or significance. Do not assume information that is not provided. Please print or write legibly.

T.G. is a 40-year-old woman who was admitted to your CCU with a positive anterior wall - MI secondary to cocaine use. Upon arrival in the unit, she still has the nitroglycerine (NTG) drip infusing that had been started in the ambulance and maintained in the ED. You are instructed to titrate the drip for relief of her chest pain. Her maintenance IV is $D_5 \frac{1}{2}$ NS at 100 ml/h. Oxygen by nasal cannula is to be titrated to keep her O_2 sat >90%. As you assess her, you find that the NTG has relieved her chest and L arm pain, but that a dull chest pressure persists and that her chest is tender to pressure. Her cardiovascular and pulmonary assessments are otherwise normal. She has a headache and is drowsy, but alert and oriented. Admission VS are 136/97, 79, 20, 37.2°C. Weight 222 pounds; height 5'2".

The report from the ED nurse is as follows: "T.G. is a single woman supporting her 3 children by working as a clerk in a small grocery store. The family is on Medicaid and lives with T.G.'s boyfriend. She has smoked 1½ packs of cigarettes a day for 15 years and has chronic hepatitis B. She also has an 18-year history of cocaine and IV heroin addiction. When using heroin, she injects the drug 2 to 3 times per day. Last night she administered the cocaine by intravenous injection for the first time in an attempt to 'stop the heroin habit.' She felt all right when she went to bed just before midnight, but woke about 0500 with severe chest pain radiating to her L arm and hand, neck, and both sides of her jaw. She also had nausea, vomiting, shortness of breath, diaphoresis, and dizziness. Her boyfriend called 911 and she was taken to the hospital by ambulance."

1. What nursing diagnoses would you choose for T.G.? List your 3 top priority diagnoses and evidence for the need for each.

Note: Obesity indicates only *energy* intake greater than body requirements. Patients presenting as obese effect have nutritional imbalances and deficits, particularly low-income patients or substance abusers who frequently have significant nutritional problems. Finally, body weight alone tells nearly nothing about nutritional status.

You look up the effects of cocaine and find that the 2 primary acute effects on the cardiovascular system are (1) blocking of the reuptake of catecholamines, resulting in increased stimulation of both alpha-adrenergic receptors (vasoconstriction) and beta-adrenergic receptors (increased heart rate and increased cardiac automaticity); and (2) blocking of the fast-sodium channel in the myocardium, resulting in depression of depolarization and a slowing of conduction velocity (local anesthetic effect). In addition, myocardial contractility is suppressed. Chronic cocaine leads to acceleration of atherosclerosis and increased tendency for platelet aggregation.

2.   Based on this information, what possible ECG changes due to cocaine toxicity would you monitor for?

3.   What physiologic complications of cocaine toxicity would you monitor for? Identify 3.

4.   Review the data on the effects of cocaine above. Propose mechanisms by which cocaine might lead to myocardial infarction.

5.   Two days after she was admitted, T.G. began to appear anxious, depressed, restless, and irritable. She is doubled over and complains of abdominal cramping. You also notice new muscle twitching and tremors. She refuses to eat. To what do you attribute these symptoms?

6.   The physician ordered methadone 10 mg PO tid for T.G. What is the rationale for prescribing methadone in this instance?

7.   Before T.G. is transferred to the telemetry floor, you consult with the social worker to identify her discharge needs. Together you list 3.

8. Shortly after T.G. is moved back to your telemetry unit, you find her disconnected telemetry unit and leads on her bed and she is nowhere to be found. When she returns about an hour later, she is very mellow and easy-going, almost lethargic. She immediately falls asleep and is difficult to arouse. To what do you attribute her absence and her present behavior?

Note: Nearly every large hospital in the country is covered by one or more drug dealers. Hospital personnel and patients who are abusing drugs need their "fix" or "hit" and are willing to pay well for it. Drug dealers are willing to oblige with personalized service.

9. What is going to be your response to the above situation?

Case Study 14

Name: _____ Class/Group: _____ Date: _____

Instructions: All questions apply to this case study. Your response should be brief and to the point. Adequate space has been provided for answers. When asked to provide several answers, they should be listed in order of priority or significance. Do not assume information that is not provided. Please print or write legibly.

You are working in the internal medicine clinic of a large teaching hospital. Today your first patient is 70-year-old J.M., a man who has been coming to the clinic for several years for management of CAD, hypertension, and anemia. A cardiac catheterization done a year ago showed 50% occlusion of the circumflex coronary artery. He has had episodes of dizziness for the past 6 months and orthostatic hypotension, shoulder discomfort, and decreased exercise tolerance for the past 2 months. On his last clinic visit 3 weeks ago, a chest x-ray and 12-lead ECG were done, showing cardiomegaly and a L bundle branch block. Results of blood studies drawn at this time were chemistries: Na 136 mEq/L, K 5.2 mEq/L, BUN 15 mg/dl, creatinine 1.8 mg/dl, glucose 82 mg/dl, and Cl 95 mEq/L. CBC: WBC 4.4 mm^3, Hgb 10.5 g/dl, Hct 31.4%, and platelets 229 mm^3. This morning his daughter has brought him to the clinic because he has had increased fatigue, significant swelling of his ankles, and shortness of breath for the last 2 days. His VS are 142/83, 105, 18, and 36.6°C.

1. Knowing his history and seeing his condition this morning, what further questions are you going to ask J.M. and his daughter?

J.M. tells you he becomes exhausted and short-of-breath climbing the stairs to his bedroom and has to lie down and rest ("put my feet up") at least an hour twice a day. He has been sleeping on 2 pillows for the last 2 weeks. He has not salted his food since the doctor told him not to because of his high blood pressure. But he admits having had peanuts and ham 3 days ago. He denies having palpitations but has had a constant, irritating, nonproductive cough lately.

2. You think it likely that J.M. has congestive heart failure. From his history, what do you identify as probable causes for his CHF?

3.   You are now ready to do your physical assessment. List at least 9 things you would assess to confirm your suspicion about the CHF. Also indicate with an "L" or an "R" whether the sign is due to left-sided or right-sided heart failure or both.

4.   The doctor confirms your feelings that J.M. is experiencing some CHF. What classes of medications might the doctor prescribe?

Note: The Hgb and Hct might be falsly decreased because of hemodilution of the CHF.

5.   This is J.M.'s first episode of significant CHF. Before he leaves the clinic you want to teach him about lifestyle modifications he can make and monitoring techniques he can use to prevent or minimize future problems. List 5 suggestions you might make and the rationale for each.

6. You tell J.M. the peanuts and ham he had 3 days ago probably set off his present episode of CHF. He looks surprised. J.M. says, "But I didn't add any salt to them!" What health care professional could he be referred to help him understand how to prevent future crises? State your rationale.

7. J.M. receives a prescription for furosemide with a potassium supplement. He wrinkles his nose at the suggestion of potassium and tells you he "hates those horse pills." He tells you a friend of his said he could eat bananas, instead. He says he would rather eat a banana everyday than take one of those pills. How will you respond?

8. It's winter and today it's 15°F. J.M. tells you he's been getting cold feet lately. This has never bothered him before. What would you suggest as comfort and safety measures?

9. Researchers sometimes call the legs "the second heart." In view of this statement and J.M.'s cardiac history, explain why "walking would be better than standing" for his circulation.

Case Study 15

J.M. is a 70-year-old retired construction worker who has experienced epigastric pain, nausea, and upset stomach for the past 6 months. He has a history of CHF, atrial fibrillation, dyspnea, hypertension, and depression, and he is on supplemental oxygen at night for sleep apnea. J.M. has just been admitted to the hospital for surgical repair of a 6.2 cm abdominal aortic aneurysm (AAA), which is now causing him constant pain. Upon arrival on your floor his VS are 109/81, 61, 16 and 98.3°F. When you perform your assessment, you find that his apical heart rhythm is irregularly irregular and his peripheral pulses are strong. His lungs are clear, and he is alert and oriented. Except for the atrial fibrillation, there are no abnormal physical findings; however, he has not had a bowel movement for 3 days. His electrolytes and other blood chemistries and clotting studies are within normal range, but his Hct is 30.1% and Hgb 9.0 g/dl.

J.M. has been depressed since the death of his wife 9 years ago. He has no children. His height is 6'2" and weight 210 pounds. His chronic medical problems have been managed over the years by medications: captopril 25 mg PO tid, digoxin 0.25 mg PO qd, fluoxetine (Prozac) 40 mg PO qd, furosemide (Lasix) 40 mg PO qd, trazodone 50 mg PO qhs, KCl 20 mEq PO bid, and lovastatin 20 mg PO bid.

1. J.M. has several common risk factors for AAA, which are evident from his health history. Identify and explain 3 factors.

2. Pain is the most common symptom of AAA. J.M.'s epigastric pain, accompanied by nausea, is typical. List 2 other common signs/symptoms of AAA that J.M. did not have and explain their significance.

While J.M. awaits his surgery, it is important that you monitor him carefully for decrease in tissue perfusion.

3. Identify 5 things you would you would be sure to assess, and state your rationale for each.

4. What is the most serious, life-threatening complication of AAA and why?

The resection of J.M.'s aneurysm was successful, but for the first 3 postop days he was delirious and required one-to-one nursing care and soft restraints before he became coherent and oriented again. He was still somewhat confused when he was transferred back to your floor.

5. List 5 nursing diagnoses that you think are high priority for J.M.'s postoperative care.

6. Postoperative care of the patient undergoing aneurysectomy includes preservation of the graft, preservation of tissue perfusion, and prevention of infection. List 3 nursing interventions that would address these issues and explain each.

When J.M. is being prepared for discharge, you talk to him about health promotion and lifestyle change issues that are pertinent for him.

7. Identify 4 health-related issues you might appropriately address with him and what you would teach in each area.

8. J.M. will be receiving follow-up visits from the home health care nurse to change his dressing and evaluate his incision. What can you do with J.M. before discharge that will help him understand what she will be doing?

Case Study 16

Name: _____ Class/Group: _____ Date: _____

Instructions: All questions apply to this case study. Your response should be brief and to the point. Adequate space has been provided for answers. When asked to provide several answers, they should be listed in order of priority or significance. Do not assume information that is not provided. Please print or write legibly.

J.C., a 40-year-old married college professor, has just been admitted to your telemetry floor with a diagnosis of "benign ventricular ectopy." He suddenly began experiencing frequent episodes of palpitations 2 years ago. These were accompanied by lightheadedness, weakness, dizziness, and decreased ability to concentrate. Holter monitoring revealed very frequent PVCs exacerbated by caffeine and exertion. On admission, he appears trim, muscular, and physically fit. As you are assessing him, he tells you that he played football in college and has lived a very active lifestyle ever since. He confides that his symptoms seriously interfere with his activities and his marital relationship, and cause him a lot of anxiety and depression, to the point where he almost "took his life" a year ago. He has been taking clonazepam (Klonopin) for his anxiety for about 18 months. His physician tried 4 different beta-blockers and the antidysrhythmic drug, mexiletine (Mexitil), to control his PVCs, but none was successful and all had unpleasant side effects. In desperation, J.C. has agreed to try another antidysrhythmic, flecainide (Tambocor), and was admitted for cardiac monitoring. His physical assessment, laboratory values, and cardiac catheterization were normal in all areas.

1.   Identify 4 relevant nursing diagnoses for J.C.

2.   Of the above problems, which is potentially life-threatening?

3.   When the heart threatens to stop working without notice, there is an understandably incredible feeling of loss of control and panic. The first objective should be to restore some sense of control to J.C. What are 5 things you could do to help relieve some of his anxiety?

4.   Review each of the following admit orders. If the order is appropriate, place an "A" in the space provided. If it is inappropriate, specify why and correct it.
___ Continuous telemetry monitoring.

___ Routine VS.

___ Activity ad lib.

___ Cardiac enzymes on admission and q8h x 3 then q AM.

___ NTG 1 0.4 mg SL prn chest pain.

___ Call physician for PVCs >6/min.

___ Low-cholesterol diet.

___ IV lock.

___ Chem 27, CBC in AM.

___ 12-lead ECG q AM.

___ Lasix 40 mg PO qd.

___ Monitor flecainide level as appropriate.

5.   List 3 appropriate nursing interventions related to J.C.'s dysrhythmia.

J.C. has just returned to his room from an exercise session in the cardiac rehab room when he collapses on the floor. You witness his fall.

6.   What are the appropriate emergency actions that you should take?

According to the cardiac monitor, J.C.'s collapse was due to a sudden episode of ventricular fibrillation. Thanks to a quick response by the hospital's CODE Team, he was successfully defibrillated and resuscitated, then transferred to the CCU (coronary care unit).

7.   What important information would you include in your report to the CCU nurse who will be caring for J.C.?

You approach J.C. saying "I think we should notify your wife about your condition." J.C. tells you she is out-of-town on a business trip but calls in regularly for messages. He asks you to call her. Note, that if he were unconscious or cognitively impaired, you *must* notify her since she is the next of kin.

8. J.C.'s wife receives the CCU nurse's message on her answering machine to call the unit. When she returns the call, what information should the nurse tell her?

9. She hisses into the telephone "What the heck do you expect *me* to do about it. There's no way I'm going to drop a good business deal to run home and hold his hand. He's sure got *you* fooled....there's nothing wrong with him that a good psychiatrist couldn't fix." As the nurse, how should you respond?

Note: In some places, the physician would make this call.

10. After J.C.'s condition has stabilized, he is referred to the cardiac rehabilitation and prevention program for an exercise prescription. A clinical exercise physiologist helps him develop individualized guidelines for safe exercise. Identify and explain the major components of an exercise prescription.

11. J.C. is used to a much more "macho" approach to exercise: "No pain, no gain." What would be the advantage to him in following an individualized plan drawn up by the exercise physiologist?

The flecainide did not work for J.C. He suffered 3 more significant episodes of ventricular fibrillation over the next 2 months and had to be defibrillated. It was decided that he would receive an implantable cardioverter defibrillator (ICD).

12. Briefly describe what an ICD is and how it works.

13. If a patient with an ICD collapsed in the shower on your unit, what safety precautions would you take before assisting him/her?

Case Study 17

Your patient, 60-year-old K.W., has a significant cardiac history. He has long-standing coronary artery disease (CAD) with occasional episodes of congestive heart failure (CHF). One year ago he had an anterior wall MI. In addition, he has chronic anemia, hypertension, chronic renal insufficiency, and a recently diagnosed 4-cm suprarenal abdominal aortic aneurysm. Because of his severe CAD, he had to retire from his job as a railroad engineer about 6 months ago. This morning he is being admitted to your telemetry unit for a same-day cardiac catheterization. As you take his health history, you note that his wife died a year ago (about the same time that he had his MI) and that he does not have any children. He is a current cigarette smoker with a 50-pack/year smoking history. As you talk with him, you realize that he has only minimal understanding of the catheterization procedure. His VS are 158/94, 88, 20 and 36.2°C.

1. Before he leaves for the cath lab, you briefly teach him the important things he needs to know before having the procedure. List 5 priority topics you will address.

Several hours later, K.W. returns from his catheterization. The cath report shows 90% occlusion of the proximal left anterior descending coronary artery (LAD), 90% occlusion of the distal LAD, 70% to 80% occlusion of the distal right coronary artery, an old apical infarct, and an ejection fraction of 37%. About an hour after the procedure was finished, you perform a brief physical assessment and find that he now has a carotid bruit, a grade III/VI systolic ejection murmur at the cardiac apex, crackles bilaterally in the lung bases, and trace pitting edema of his feet and ankles. Except for a soft systolic murmur, these findings were not present before the catheterization.

2. What is your evaluation of the catheterization results?

3. What problem do the changes in assessment findings suggest to you and identify what led you to your conclusion?

4.   List 4 actions you would take as a result of your evaluation of the assessment and state your rationales.

After assessing the patient, K.W.'s doctor admitted him with a diagnosis of CAD and CHF for coronary artery bypass graft (CABG) surgery. Significant lab results drawn at this time were Hct 25.3%, Hgb 8.8 g/dl, BUN 33 mg/dl and creatinine 3.1 mg/dl. K.W. was diuresed with Lasix and given 2 units of packed red blood cells (PRBCs).

5.   Review K.W.'s health history. Can you identify a probable explanation for his chronic renal insufficiency and anemia?

Five days later, after his condition was stabilized, K.W. was taken to surgery for bypass of 3 coronary arteries (CABG x 3). When he arrived in the SICU he had a Swan-Ganz catheter in place for hemodynamic monitoring and was intubated and on a ventilator at FIO_2 .70 and PEEP 5 cm H_2O. His first hemodynamic readings were: pulmonary artery pressure (PAP) 41/23 mm Hg, CVP 13 mm Hg, PCWP 13 mm Hg, cardiac index (CI) 1.88 L/min/m^2. ABGs drawn at this time were: pH 7.36, PCO_2 46 mm Hg, PO_2 61 mm Hg, and SaO_2 85%, with a Hgb 10.3 mg/dl.

6.   What is your evaluation of his hemodynamic status based on the above parameters?

Clinically, these values show that the pressures within his heart and lungs are a little high and that his cardiac output is a little low, indicating that his heart is still having difficulty pumping out all the blood that is returned to it and/or that he is a little fluid overloaded. His condition will require careful monitoring.

7.   K.W. is receiving continuous IV infusions of nitroprusside (Nipride) and dobutamine (Dobutrex). He also has just received 2 units of fresh frozen plasma (FFP) and 500 ml of albumin IV. Given this information, do you think the hemodynamic values reported above reflect poor L ventricular function or fluid overload and why?

8. Why is K.W. receiving the nitroprusside and dobutamine?

9. What is your responsibility when administering nitroprusside and dobutamine to your patient?

10. Why did he receive the FFP and albumin?

11. Explain whether or not it is possible for K.W. to experience a transfusion reaction when receiving albumin or FFP infusion.

12. What is your interpretation of his ABGs on 70% O_2?

After 3 days in the SICU, K.W.s condition was stable and he was returned to your telemetry floor. Now, 5 days later, he is ready to go home, and you are preparing him for discharge.

13. List at least 5 general areas related to his CABG surgery in which he should receive instruction before he goes home.

Case Study 18

Name: _____ Class/Group: _____ Date: _____

Instructions: All questions apply to this case study. Your response should be brief and to the point. Adequate space has been provided for answers. When asked to provide several answers, they should be listed in order of priority or significance. Do not assume information that is not provided. Please print or write legibly.

It is midmorning on the cardiac unit where you work and you are getting a new patient, G.P. G.P., a 60-year-old retired businessman, is married and has 3 grown children. As you take his health history, he tells you that he began feeling changes in his heart rhythm about 10 days ago. He has hypertension and a 10-year history of angina pectoris. During the past week he has had more frequent episodes of midchest discomfort. The chest pain has awakened him from sleep but does respond to NTG, which he has taken sublingually about 8 to 10 times over the past week. During the week he has also experienced increased fatigue. He states, "I have lost my sensation of well-being." A cardiac catheterization done several years ago revealed 50% occlusion of the right coronary artery (RCA) and 50% occlusion of the left anterior descending (LAD) coronary artery. He tells you that both his mother and father had CAD. He is taking amlodipine and metoprolol.

1. What other information are you going to ask about his episodes of chest pain?

2. What are common sites for radiation of ischemic cardiac pain?

3. You know that G.P. has atherosclerosis of the coronary arteries but he has not told you about his risk factors. You need to know his risk factors for CAD in order to plan teaching for lifestyle modifications. What questions will you ask him?

4. Although he has been taking SL NTG for a long time, you want to be sure he is using it correctly. What information would you make sure he understands about the side effects, use, and storage of sublingual NTG?

When you first admitted G.P., you placed him on telemetry and observed he was in atrial fibrillation converting frequently to atrial flutter with a 4:1 block. His VS and all of his lab tests were within normal range, including LDH and CPK levels; K was 4.7 mEq/L. He was converted with medications (quinidine and diltiazem) from atrial fib/flutter to tachy/brady syndrome with long sinus pauses that caused lightheadedness and hypotension.

5. What risks does the new rhythm pose for G.P.?

Because G.P.'s dysrhythmia was causing unacceptable symptoms, he was taken to surgery and a permanent DDI pacemaker was placed and set at a rate of 70/minute.

6. What does the code "DDI" mean?

7. The pacemaker insertion surgery places G.P. at risk for several serious complications. List 3 potential problems that you will monitor for as you care for him.

8. G.P. will need some education regarding his new pacemaker. What information will you give him before he leaves the hospital?

Note: Information about the Medic Alert emergency identification system can be obtained by calling 1-800-432-5378.

9. G.P.'s wife approaches you and anxiously inquires, "My neighbor saw this science fiction movie about this guy who got a pacemaker and then he couldn't die. Is that for real?" How are you going to respond to her?

After discharge, G.P. is referred to a cardiac prevention and rehabilitation center to start an exercise program. He will be exercise tested, and an individualized exercise prescription will be developed for him based on the exercise test.

   10. What information will be obtained from the graded exercise (stress) test (GXT) and what is included in an exercise prescription?

Case Study 19

Name: _____ Class/Group: _____ Date: _____

Instructions: All questions apply to this case study. Your response should be brief and to the point. Adequate space has been provided for answers. When asked to provide several answers, they should be listed in order of priority or significance. Do not assume information that is not provided. Please print or write legibly.

C.W., a 70-year-old man, was brought to the ED at 0430 this morning by his wife. She told the ED triage nurse that he had dysentery for the past 3 days and last night he had a lot of "dark red" diarrhea. When he became very dizzy, disoriented, and weak this morning, she decided to bring him to the hospital. C.W.'s VS were systolic BP 70 mm Hg, diastolic BP inaudible (70/-); 110, 20. A 16-gauge IV catheter was inserted and a LR infusion was started. The triage nurse obtained the following history from the patient and his wife. C.W. has had idiopathic dilated cardiomyopathy (IDCM) for several years. The onset was insidious but the cardiomyopathy is now severe, as evidenced by a L ventricular ejection fraction of 13% found during a recent cardiac catheterization. He experiences frequent problems with CHF because of the IDCM. Two years ago he had a cardiac arrest that was attributed to hypokalemia. He also has a long history of hypertension and arthritis. Fifteen years ago he had a peptic ulcer.

An endoscopy showed a 25 x 15 mm duodenal ulcer with adherent clot. The ulcer was cauterized and C.W. was admitted to the MICU for treatment of his volume deficit. You are his admitting nurse. As you are making him comfortable, Mrs. W. gives you a paper sack filled with the bottles of medications he has been taking: enalopril (Vasotec) 5 mg PO bid, warfarin (Coumadin) 2 mg PO qd, digoxin 0.125 mg PO qd, KCl 20 mEq PO bid, and tolmetin (an NSAID) 400 mg PO tid. As you connect him to the cardiac monitor, you note that he is in atrial fibrillation. Doing a quick assessment, you find a pale man who is sleepy but arousable and oriented. He is still dizzy, hypotensive, and tachycardic. You hear S_3 and S_4 heart sounds and a grade II/VI systolic murmur. Peripheral pulses are all 2+ and trace pedal edema is present. Lungs are clear. Bowel sounds are present, midepigastric tenderness is noted, and the liver margin is 4 cm below the costal margin. A Swan-Ganz catheter and an arterial line are inserted.

1. What medications probably precipitated C.W.'s GI bleeding?

2. What is the most serious potential complication of C.W.'s bleeding?

3. From his history and assessment, identify 5 signs/symptoms (direct and/or indirect) of GI bleeding and loss of blood volume.

C.W. received a total of 8 units of PRBCs, 5 units of fresh frozen plasma (FFP), and many liters of crystalloids to keep his systolic BP above 90 mm Hg. On the second day in the MICU, his total fluid intake was 8.498 L and output 3.660 L for a positive fluid balance of 4.838 L. His hemodynamic parameters after fluid resuscitation were PCWP 30 mm Hg, cardiac output 4.5 L/min.

4.   Why will you want to monitor his fluid status very carefully?

5.   List 6 things you will monitor to assess C.W.'s fluid balance.

6.   Explain the purpose of the fresh frozen plasma for C.W.

As soon as you get a chance, you look at his admission lab results. The K is 6.2 mEq/L, BUN 90 mg/dl, creatinine 2.1 mg/dl, Hgb 8.4 g/dl, Hct 25%, WBC 16 mm^3, and PT 18.3 sec. Other results are within the normal range.

7.   Are you worried by the elevated K? Why, or why not? Explain your answer.

8.   Why do you think BUN and creatinine are elevated?

9.   What do the low Hb and Hct levels indicate about the rapidity of his blood loss?

10. What is the explanation for the prolonged PT?

11. How do you account for the elevated WBC count?

Mrs. W. has been with her husband since he arrived at the ED and is very worried about his condition and his care.

12. List 4 things you might do to make her more comfortable while her husband is in the MICU.

Case Study 20

K.K., a 40-year-old administrative secretary, lost consciousness and slumped to the floor while eating dinner with her husband. He initiated CPR. Paramedics arrived within 4 to 5 minutes and found her in ventricular fibrillation. After successful defibrillation, she was transported to the hospital. In the MICU her nurse obtained K.K.'s health history from her husband. She has a long history of RHD (rheumatic heart disease) with MVP (mitral valve prolapse) and severe L ventricular dysfunction. She has had atrial fibrillation/atrial flutter for 6 years. She also has had ventricular dysrhythmias for several years being treated with various antidysrhythmic drugs; furosemide, however, she was not taking her medications at the time of the arrest because of their unpleasant side effects. Her doctor feels she has been noncompliant with her medications and that she is denying her need for mitral valve replacement. For the past 2 months she has had CHF with greatly decreased activity tolerance. Medications she was taking at the time of the arrest were: furosemide (Lasix) 80 mg PO qd, KCl 20 mEq PO bid, digoxin 0.125 mg PO qd, lisinopril (Zestril) 5 mg PO qd, verapamil (Verelan) 120 mg PO qd, and warfarin (Coumadin) 2.5 mg PO qd. On the day of her arrest she had diarrhea.

1. From K.K.'s history, what factors probably contributed to her cardiac arrest?

On admission to the MICU, K.K. was hypotensive and unresponsive to voice commands. She was intubated and placed on mechanical ventilation. A central line was inserted, and dopamine and lidocaine drips started. For the first day in the MICU she remained unresponsive to commands, pupillary reaction was sluggish, eyes deviated slowly to the right, upper extremities had increased tone, and lower extremities were flaccid. Painful stimuli elicited withdrawal and decorticate posturing. Her 12-lead ECG showed atrial fibrillation at a rate of 136/min, ST segment depression in leads II, III, AVF and V_1-V_6 and T wave inversion in leads V_3-V_5.

2. What is the probable cause for her neurologic deficits?

3. Explain how rapid atrial fibrillation can cause a decrease in cardiac output and contribute to CHF.

4.   What is the significance of the ST segment depression and T wave inversion in her 12-lead ECG?

5.   List 8 lab results that the MICU nurse should check as soon as possible.

After 4 days in the MICU, K.K.'s condition was stabilized and she was transferred to your telemetry floor. When you first assess her, you find jugular vein distention at 10 cm and hear a grade II/VI systolic murmur and an S_3 sound. A thrill is felt over the precordium, and the S_1 and S_2 can be seen on the chest. She no longer has sensory or motor deficits, and her long-term memory is good. However, she is confused, oriented only to name, and has poor short-term memory. Her lidocaine level in the MICU the day before the transfer (the day the lidocaine was discontinued) was 16.8 mg/L; digoxin level was normal. A cardiac catheterization and ECHO cardiogram showed that K.K. has irreversible heart valve, L ventricle, and L atrium damage and is no longer a candidate for mitral valve replacement. She states she is very fearful about her memory loss and the inoperable heart damage.

6.   List 3 factors that might be contributing to K.K.'s confusion and disorientation.

7.   List 4 nursing interventions you might implement to relieve K.K.'s fear.

After 2 weeks in the hospital, K.K. is scheduled for placement of an internal cardioverter defibrillator (ICD) to prevent future cardiac arrest from ventricular fibrillation. You will do her preoperative teaching about ICDs.

8.   What is an ICD and how does it work?

9.   List 4 discharge instructions related to the ICD that you will give K.K.

Case Study 21

During a routine checkup, D.A.'s doctor heard 2 new heart murmurs: a grade II/VI diastolic flow murmur heard at the R sternal border and a prominent grade IV/VI systolic ejection murmur heard over the entire precordium but best at the L sternal border. The murmurs are asymptomatic. D.A. is a slender, active 50-year-old engineer, married with 2 teenage children. He has polycystic kidney disease with renal failure and has been on dialysis for 5 years. His mother also had polycystic kidney disease. Besides frequent UTIs, he has no other significant medical problems, no history of cardiac disease, and no cardiac risk factors. A transthoracic/transesophageal ECHO showed a "high pressure jet from the R atrium or R ventricle." Cardiac catheterization showed an "aortic to R ventricle connection through a R coronary sinus of Valsalva leak." The catheterization also showed normal coronary arteries, normal L ventricular function, and no aortic regurgitation.

D.A. was admitted to the hospital for surgical repair of a ruptured sinus of Valsalva aneurysm. During the surgery a 4-mm hole from the R coronary sinus to the R atrium was discovered and repaired with a patch. There were no complication. You are caring for D.A. in the SICU after the surgery. On the first postop day his VS are 90/54, 87, 12, 37.8°C. Central venous pressure averages 10 mm Hg. He has a temporary pacemaker set at 87/min, which is functioning correctly. Lungs are clear. He has been extubated and is on O_2 at 2 L/min by nasal cannula with an SaO_2 of 99%. He has a chest tube and indwelling urinary catheter. You review his lab results, noting BUN 120 mg/dl, creatinine 8.5 mg/dl, and K 6.2 mEq/L. His preop Hct was 32%; today it is 22.1% and Hgb is 9.0 g/dL. Other lab values are within normal ranges.

1.   Which of the physiologic data reported above should cause you concern and prompt careful monitoring on your part?

2.   When you perform your physical assessment, you should pay special attention to signs/symptoms related to D.A.'s problems. List at least 5 priority assessment areas, and explain why they are important.

3. Mrs. A. is present at the bedside, supportive and anxious. Considering her apprehension, what can you do to make her more comfortable?

On the third postop day, D.A. had an infectious disease consult. The consulting physician wrote in the chart, "The *Enterobacter* infection of the sinus of Valsalva is the likely cause of the aneurysm. The heart was probably seeded from a renal source. If the patch continues to harbor organisms, the patient may have future problems." D.A. was started on IV antibiotics (gentamicin, ticarcillin, and cefuroxime [Zinacef]).

4. List at least 3 problems D.A. might have as a result of the heavy-duty antibiotic therapy. What will you monitor for each? Consider his renal failure and common side effects of the medications.

5. Mrs. A. confides in you, "You know, my 15-year-old son refuses to talk about his dad's illness. He won't even come to see him in the hospital. The guidance counselor called from school yesterday and said he's been acting out in school. I'm exhausted trying to work family life from both ends." How are you going to respond?

6. In preparation for discharge, a peripherally inserted central catheter (PICC) is placed. What is a PICC, and what are the advantages and disadvantages of this type of catheter?

D.A. is being discharged to home, where a home care nurse will continue to monitor the IV site and teach the wife how to administer the IV antibiotics.

7.   Identify 2 nursing diagnosis that would apply to IV antibiotic administration in the home?

Case Study 22

Name: _____ Class/Group: _____ Date: _____

Instructions: All questions apply to this case study. Your response should be brief and to the point. Adequate space has been provided for answers. When asked to provide several answers, they should be listed in order of priority or significance. Do not assume information that is not provided. Please print or write legibly.

You are in the middle of your shift in the CCU of a large urban medical center. Your new admission, C.B., a 47-year-old woman, has just been brought by Life Flight to your institution from a small rural community over 100 miles away. She is unstable after an acute MI. C.B.'s VS are 100/60, 86, 14. After you make C.B. comfortable, you receive this report from the AirMed nurse: "C.B. is a full-time homemaker with 4 children. She has had episodes of 'chest tightness' for several years but this is her first documented MI. She has elevated cholesterol and triglyceride levels and has smoked 1 ½ packs of cigarettes per day for 30 years. Besides this and recent night sweats and hot flashes, she doesn't have any other medical problems. Yesterday at 2000 she began having substernal chest pain that radiated to her neck bilaterally and down both arms. She rated the pain as '9' on a scale of 1 to 10. She lay down with a heating pad but the pain didn't go away. Her husband then took her to the local ED where a 12-lead ECG showed hyperacute ST elevation. They were about to give her some t-PA when she went into V fib (ventricular fibrillation) and arrested. She was successfully defibrillated with 2 shocks. Then she was given the t-PA and put on lidocaine, heparin, and nitroglycerin drips. They also gave her some metoprol. This morning when her systolic pressure (BP) dropped into the 80s, she was put on a dopamine drip and flown here for a possible PTCA (percutaneous transluminal coronary angioplasty). Right now the lidocaine is going at 2 mg/min, the heparin at 1200 μ/h, and the dopamine at 5 μ/kg/min. The nitroglycerin is off."

The Life Flight nurse hands you a copy of yesterday's 12-lead ECG that shows normal sinus rhythm with ST elevation in leads II, III, AVF, and V_5-V_6. She also gives you a copy of yesterday's lab work: Na 145 mEq/L, K 3.6 mEq/L, HCO_3 19 mEq/L, BUN 9 mg/dl, creatinine 0.8 mg/dl, WBC 14.5 mm^3, Hct 44.3%, and Hgb 14.5 g/dl.

1.   Given her diagnosis of acute MI, what other lab results are you going to look at?

2. You found the following lab results in the patient's chart. For each, interpret the result, and evaluate the meaning for C.B.
   a. CPKs drawn upon admission to the ED and at 4 hour intervals were: 95 U/L, 1931 U/L, and 4175 U/L. CPK-MB isoenzymes were: 5%, 79%, and 216%.

   b. Cholesterol: 180 mg/dl.

   c. SaO_2 on O_2 at 6 L/min by nasal cannula: >90%.

   d. PT was 11.9 secs and PTT was 26.9 secs (before heparin infusion).

   e. Mg level was 2.2 mg/dl.

3. Why wasn't the LDH reported on the blood drawn in the ED?

4. The 12-lead ECG can tell you the location of the infarction. Look at the leads that show ST elevation (see above). What areas of C.B.'s heart have been damaged?

5. What is t-PA? Why is it given and when is it given to a patient having an MI? How is it administered?

6. An hour after her admission, you are preparing C.B. for her PTCA. Evaluate her readiness for teaching and her learning needs. What would you tell her?

The following day you care for C.B. again. During her PTCA procedure yesterday a circumflex coronary lesion was found and the artery was successfully dilated. She is still on the lidocaine and heparin drips. The dopamine has been discontinued. VS are stable. PCWP is 20 mm Hg and cardiac output is 7.3 L/min. You check her lab results for lidocaine and PTT levels.

7.   The lidocaine level is 2.5 μg/ml, and the PTT is 61 seconds. Analyze the results and state any actions you would take.

As you work with C.B., you notice that she is extremely anxious. You had observed some anxiety yesterday which you had attributed to the strange CCU environment, pain, and anticipation of the PTCA procedure. You know that the PTCA was successful and that she is physically stable. You wonder what is wrong. She tells you that her MI occurred right in the middle of a move with her family from her rural community to an even smaller and unfamiliar town some 500 miles away in a neighboring state. She is dreading the move. Her husband "becomes angry easily and starts lashing out" toward her and the children. She is afraid to move to a community where she will have no friends and family to support her.

8.   How can you help your patient? Evaluate the situation and describe possible interventions.

9.   C.B.'s husband comes to visit. He is a handsome, well-dressed man who appears to be loving and attentive toward C.B. He brought a bouquet of roses for her and a box of chocolates for the nurses, "Because I appreciate how good you girls have been to my wife." One of your younger colleagues comments to you, "Why, what a nice guy! What is her problem? Every woman would love to be married to a man like that!" How are you going to respond?

CHAPTER 2: PULMONARY DISORDERS

Case Study 1

Name: _____ Class/Group: _____ Date: _____

Instructions: All questions apply to this case study. Your response should be brief and to the point. Adequate space has been provided for answers. When asked to provide several answers, they should be listed in order of priority or significance. Do not assume information that is not provided. Please print or write legibly.

A.K. is a 38-year-old woman who runs 3 miles every morning. She comes to the Family Nurse Practitioner Clinic with complaints of a burning feeling in her throat and upper airway that begins shortly after she starts running. She states that she gets increasingly more winded and sometimes has to stop running to catch her breath.

1. As the intake nurse working in the clinic, what routine information would you want to obtain from A.K.?

2. What two body systems do you suspect might be involved in A.K.'s problem?

3. What would you do to differentiate between problems in the two body systems?

You assess A.K. and note the following: S_1S_2 with no murmurs, clicks, or rubs; on inspiration her heart rate speeds up and you think you hear a split S_2; and on expiration her heart rate slows down and you don't hear the split.

4. Discuss the significance of these findings.

Her lungs are clear throughout and percuss resonance. You measure height and weight to calculate her *estimated* peak expiratory flow rate (PEFR). You then measure A.K.'s *actual* PEFR using a peak flow meter (PFM).

5. Explain the purpose of the PEFR measurement.

6. You record A.K.'s PEFR measurement and note that it is within 5% of estimated normal PEFR. Discuss the significance of her pulmonary evaluation and these findings.

The FNP confirms your examination findings and, after reviewing A.K.'s PEFR measurements, discusses the possibility of exercise-induced asthma (EIA) with A.K. She directs A.K. to record her PEFR then go for her usual morning run. If she experiences the burning feeling in her throat and upper airway and/or becomes short of breath, she should stop running and immediately measure and record her PEFR. Repeat measurements should be taken at 5 minute intervals for 20 to 30 minutes. Ask A.K. to bring her PEFR record with her next time.

7.   What is the FNP hoping to learn from the presymptom to postsymptom PEFR measurement?

A.K. returns in 1 week for a follow-up visit. She hands you a list of PEFR measurements. You calculate that A.K.'s postrun measurements range from 75% to 85% of her prerun values and her PEFR returned to normal within 25 minutes of stopping activity.

8.   What does this patterns of change indicate?

The FNP gives A.K. an albuterol (Ventolin) metered-dose inhaler (MDI) with a spacer and instructs her to take 2 puffs 15 minutes before she exercises. The FNP is called to see another patient and asks you to complete the discharge teaching with A.K.

9.   What information should you discuss with her?

10.   A.K. says she doesn't like to be dependent on medication. How would you respond to her statement?

11.   A.K. asks if it is possible for her to develop full-blown asthma. How would you respond?

A.K. was motivated to take her MDI so she could maintain her exercise regimen. At a follow-up visit, she tells you she saw, "Lots of folks using an MDI at last Saturday's race."

Case Study 2

Name: _____ Class/Group: _____ Date: _____

Instructions: All questions apply to this case study. Your response should be brief and to the point. Adequate space has been provided for answers. When asked to provide several answers, they should be listed in order of priority or significance. Do not assume information that is not provided. Please print or write legibly.

M.N., age 40, is admitted with acute cholecystitis, elevated WBC, and a fever of 102°F. She has undergone a cholecystectomy and has been transferred to your floor from ICU the second day postop. She has an NGT to continuous low wall suction, one peripheral IV, and a large abdominal dressing. Her orders are as follows: progress diet as tolerated; $D_5\frac{1}{4}$ NS with 40 mEq KCl at 125 ml an hour; turn, cough, and deep breathe q2h; incentive spirometer (IS) q2h while awake; dangle in AM, ambulate in PM; morphine sulfate 10 mg IM q4h for pain; ampicillin (Omnipen) 2 g IVPB q6h; chest x-ray (CXR) in AM.

1. Are these orders appropriate for M.N.? State your rationale.

2. Identify the two most common respiratory-related complications for patients with abdominal or thoracic surgery.

3. What information and assessments would help you differentiate between the two complications in Question 2?

4. What procedure is necessary to differentiate between atelectasis and pneumonia?

5. You are assigned to take care of M.N. Her VS are 148/82, 118, 24, 101°F. Her SaO_2 is 88%. Based on these numbers, what do you think is going on with M.N. and why?

6. You know M.N. is at risk for postop atelectasis. What is atelectasis?

After morning report you do an assessment and auscultate decreased breath sounds and crackles in the R base posteriorly. Her RML and RLL percuss slightly dull. She splints her R side when attempting to take a deep breath. You suspect that she is developing atelectasis.

7.   What most likely accounts for M.N.'s inspiratory-related behavior?

8.   What effect will M.N.'s splinting have on potential atelectasis?

9.   Identify and clarify 5 actions you would take next.

10.   What 4 interventions might be used for pulmonary hygiene?

11.   Identify 3 outcomes that you expect for M.N. as a result of pulmonary hygiene and increased activity?

12.   M.N.'s sister questions you, saying, "I don't understand. She came in here with a bad gallbladder. What has happened to her lungs?" How would you respond?

13.   Radiology calls up with a report from the radiologist on the AM CXR. M.N. has atelectasis. Will that change anything from what you have already planned for M.N.? Explain what you would do differently if M.N. had pneumonia.

Case Study 3

Name: _____ *Class/Group:* _____ *Date:* _____

Instructions: All questions apply to this case study. Your response should be brief and to the point. Adequate space has been provided for answers. When asked to provide several answers, they should be listed in order of priority or significance. Do not assume information that is not provided. Please print or write legibly.

You are a public health nurse working at a county immunization and TB clinic. B.A. is a 61-year-old woman who wishes to obtain a food handler's license and is required to show proof of a negative Mantoux (PPD) test before being hired. She came to your clinic 2 days ago to obtain a PPD test for tuberculosis. She has returned to have you evaluate her reaction.

1. The CDC recommends screening people at high risk for TB and provide preventive therapy for those at high risk for developing active disease. What populations are at high risk?

2. What is the preferred method for TB screening?

3. When should the individual return to have the test interpreted?

4. How do you determine if the test is positive or negative?

Note: The American Thoracic Society and Center for Disease Control have adopted the following guidelines for positive Mantoux reaction:
  - A PPD induration ≥ 5 mm is considered positive for persons with or at-risk for HIV infection; those who have had close, recent contact with someone who has infectious tuberculosis; or persons who have CXR that show old, healed TB.
  - A PPD induration ≥ 10 mm is considered positive for foreign-born persons from high prevalence countries; IV drug users; medically underserved, low income populations; residents of long-term care facilities; people with chronic illnesses; and all children and adolescents.
  - A PPD induration ≥ 15 mm is considered positive for all other persons.

5. What additional information would you want to obtain from B.A. before interpreting her skin test result as positive or negative?

Although B.A. was reluctant to give information, she stated that she was exposed to TB as a child, acknowledges consuming 3 to 4 oz ETOH/day, and has smoked 1 ½ packs per day for 40 years. She lives with her daughter and becomes angry at the suggestion that she might have TB.

6.   Three days later, you measure B.A.'s skin test and note that the area of erythema measures 30 mm in diameter and the area of hardness measures 20 mm in diameter. Determine if B.A.'s skin test is positive or negative.

7.   What does a positive PPD result mean?

8.   How would you determine if someone like B.A. has active tuberculosis?

The physician in your TB clinic determines that B.A.'s CXR is clear (shows no signs of any TB). The CDC recommends preventive therapy for adults with evidence of infection but no active disease.

9.   According to the American Thoracic Society/Centers for Disease Control (1990) guidelines, what constitutes usual preventive therapy?

10.   What is the age-related side effect of preventive therapy?

11.   Based on the information B.A. gave about her history, identify what public health follow-up would be warranted?

Because of her age, ETOH consumption, negative CXR, and resistance to discussing TB, the physician decides not to discuss the option of preventive therapy with B.A.

12.   What information should B.A. receive before leaving the clinic?

B.A. was hired under the condition that she must immediately report any signs and/or symptoms of active disease to the county health department or her physician and have a yearly CXR.

Case Study 4

P.R., a 31-year-old woman, contracted an upper respiratory tract infection, developed a high fever, and began to experience progressive ascending paralysis. She was admitted to the local hospital, diagnosed with Guillain-Barré syndrome, and 10 days later was discharged to home with home health care nurses, from your agency, around the clock. She is intubated and mechanically ventilated. Her VS are 112/68, 134, 12, 101°F. The placement of her nasal-duodenal tube was confirmed by abdominal x-ray. Her total parenteral nutrition (TPN) was discontinued yesterday and she was started on enteral nutrition (EN). The consulting dietician calculated P.R.'s caloric need at 2800 calories/24 hours because of her fever.

1.   Identify and discuss 3 factors that would influence the physician's decision to place P.R. on EN.

2.   Absolute medical contraindications to enteral feeding (EN) are few, and it is preferable to demonstrate failure of EN than to assume that the GI tract is nonfunctional and initiate TPN. Give 3 examples of medical diagnoses for which EN would be contraindicated.

3.   Pulmonary aspiration is a risk with enteral feedings, although the risk is substantially reduced with duodenal placement. Identify 4 measures that can be taken to minimize the risk of aspiration.

4.   Identify 5 strategies for preventing bacterial contamination of the feeding formula and tubing.

5.   Identify 2 indicators that an EN infusion rate is too rapid.

6.   The nurse needs to monitor P.R.'s GI response to EN and steroid therapy. Identify 2 observations that need to be recorded, and explain the significance of each.

7.   It is a common belief that diarrhea (defined as > 3 liquid stools/day) is a natural consequence of EN administration. Discuss whether this is a true statement.

8.   Identify 3 factors that could cause diarrhea.

As P.R.'s nurse, you are concerned about meeting her needs for fluids, oral hygiene, skin integrity, and activity.

9.   Discuss 5 indicators that would help you assess fluid status.

10.   The goal related to P.R.'s mouth care is to preserve the oral mucosa and dentition. Identify 3 strategies for providing oral hygiene with an oral endotracheal tube (ETT) in place.

11.   What is the rationale for not taking an oral temperature in the vicinity of an ETT?

12.   You assess P.R.'s skin every 4 hours. Identify 3 treatment goals in relation to skin/positioning.

13.   What 4 strategies will facilitate the expected outcome of maintaining skin integrity?

14. You approach P.R. to begin ROM exercises. You ask her if she is experiencing muscle pain at this time and she nods "yes." You tell P.R. that you will wait until she is pain-free to perform the exercises. Why?

It took 4 months for P.R. to make a full recovery.

Case Study 5

Name: _____ Class/Group: _____ Date: _____

Instructions: All questions apply to this case study. Your response should be brief and to the point. Adequate space has been provided for answers. When asked to provide several answers, they should be listed in order of priority or significance. Do not assume information that is not provided. Please print or write legibly.

M.N., a 22-year-old man, is highly allergic to dust and pollen; anxiety appears to play a role in exacerbating his asthma attacks. His wife drove M.N. to the clinic when his wheezing was unresponsive to beclomethasone (Vanceril) and ipratropium bromide (Atrovent) inhalers. Upon arrival, his VS are 152/84, 124, 42, 100.4°F. M.N. is started on 4 L O_2/nc, an IV of D_5W at KVO, and ABGs were pH 7.31, $PaCO_2$ 48 mm Hg, HCO_3 26 mEq/L, PaO_2 55 mm Hg, SaO_2 86%.

1. Explain the pathophysiology of asthma.

2. Identify pathophysiologic responses during an asthma attack.

3. Are M.N.'s VS acceptable? State your rationale.

4. Identify the drug classifications and actions of Vanceril and Atrovent.

5. Are Vanceril and/or Atrovent appropriate for use during an asthma attack?

6. The physician orders albuterol 3 mg nebulization treatment STAT. What is the rationale for this order?

7. What is the rationale for immediately starting M.N. on oxygen?

8.   List 5 short-term interventions that may help relieve M.N.'s symptoms.

After several hours of IV and PO rehydration and a second albuterol treatment, M.N.'s wheezing and chest tightness resolve, and he is able to expectorate his secretions. The doctor discusses M.N.'s asthma management with him, and he tells him that his inhalers meet his needs on a day-to-day basis but fail him when he has an asthma attack. The doctor discharges M.N. with a prescription for Proventil MDI and a "spacer" and recommends that he call the pulmonary clinic for follow-up with a pulmonary specialist.

9.   What issues would you address in discharge teaching with M.N.?

You ask M.N. to demonstrate the use of his MDI. He vigorously shakes the canister, holds the aerosolizer at an angle (pointing toward his cheek) in front of his mouth, and squeezes the canister as he takes a quick, deep breath.

10.   What common mistakes has M.N. made when using the inhaler?

11.   How would you council M.N. about the use of his MDI?

12.   What is the function of a peak flow meter (PFM) and how are they used?

13.   M.N.'s wife asks about the possibility of M.N. having another attack. How would you respond?

14.   Identify 4 nursing diagnoses that apply to M.N.

Case Study 6

J.D., a 38-year-old man, is admitted to your medical floor with a diagnosis of pleural effusion. He complains of shortness of breath, pain in his chest, and weakness. His VS are 142/82, 118, 38 labored and shallow, 102°F. His chest x-ray (CXR) shows a large pleural effusion and pulmonary infiltrates in the right lower lobe (RLL) consistent with pneumonia.

1. Given his diagnosis, are J.D.'s admission vital signs expected? State your rationale.

2. What is pleural effusion?

3. List 3 common causes of pleural effusion?

4. Review the pathophysiology and consequences of pleural effusion and pulmonary infiltrates.

5. What is the difference between exudate and transudate?

6. How does the underlying pathophysiology give rise to the presenting signs and symptoms?

The physician performs a thoracentesis and drains 1500 ml fluid. A specimen for C&S is sent to the laboratory, and the patient is started on cefuroxime 1 g IVPB q8h.

7. What is a thoracentesis?

8. What maneuvers would promote the clearance of pulmonary secretions?

9. You enter the room to reposition J.D. If J.D. is supine, what side would you turn him to and why?

10. The pleural fluid C&S results indicate large amount *Klebsiella* growth that is sensitive to cefuroxime. What action should you take next?

11. Because fluid continues to collect in the pleural space, the physician decides to insert a pleural chest tube under nonemergent conditions. What is your responsibility as J.D.'s nurse?

12. Evaluate each of the following statements about chest tube drainage systems. Place a "T" (true) or "F" (false) in the space provided. Discuss why the "false" statement(s) are incorrect on the next page.
    a. ___ It is the height of the column of water in the suction control mechanism not the setting of the suction source that actually limits the amount of suction transmitted to the pleural cavity.
    b. ___ A suction pressure of +20 cm H_2O is commonly recommended for adults.
    c. ___ Bubbling in the water seal chamber means that air is leaking from the lungs, the tubing, or the insertion site.
    d. ___ The rise and fall of the water level with the patient's respirations reflects normal pressure changes in the pleural cavity with respirations.
    e. ___ The chamber is a closed system; therefore water cannot evaporate.
    f. ___ To declot the drainage tubing, put lotion on your hands, compress the tubing, and strip long segments of the tubing before releasing.
    g. ___ You lower the bed on top of the drainage system and break it. Because you noted an air leak from the lung during your initial assessment, you may clamp the chest tube for the short time it takes to reestablish the drainage system.
    h. ___ The chest tube becomes disconnected from the drainage system. Because you noted an air leak from the lung during your initial assessment, you can submerge the chest tube 1 to 2 inches below the surface of a 250 ml bottle of sterile saline or water.
    i. ___ The collection chamber is full so you need to connect a new drainage system to the chest tube. It is appropriate to momentarily clamp the chest tube while you disconnect the old system and reconnect the new.
    j. ___ The drainage system falls over, spilling the chest drainage into the other drainage columns. The total amount of drainage can be obtained by adding the amount of drainage in each of the columns.

Discussion for "false" statement(s):

13. It is visiting hours. An attractive young woman approaches you at the desk and, stating she is J.D.'s wife, asks what room he is in. You know that another woman, his real wife, is in the room with him now. How are you going to handle this?

J.D. did some fast talking and managed to avoid discovery, He received aggressive antibiotic and pulmonary therapy and was discharged 5 days later.

Case Study 7

C.E., a 73-year-old married man, visits his internist complaining that he becomes "so winded" with activity. C.E.'s pulse oximetry (SaO_2) registers 83% at rest. He is sent to the local hospital for a CXR and ABGs to be drawn after resting 20 minutes on room air. The next day, his physician calls C.E. and informs him that he has severe emphysema and must start on continuous oxygen therapy. The physician tells C.E. that his office will have a home health equipment company call him to make arrangements to deliver the equipment and educate him in its use. As an RN working for the company, you are assigned to make the initial home visit.

1. How would you prepare for the first visit?

2. What issues would you address with C.E. and his wife?

3. The next time you visit, C.E. complains about sores behind his ears. He explains, "That long oxygen tubing seems to take on a life of its own. It twists around and gets caught under doors, chairs, everything. It darn near rips the ears off my head." He asks for your help. How would you respond?

4. You auscultate C.E.'s breath sounds and detect the odor of Vicks Vapo Rub. When you question C.E. about the use of Vicks, he tells you that he started to apply it in and around his nose to prevent his nose from becoming dry and sore. How would you council C.E. and his wife?

C.E. elected to use liquid oxygen because it offers more freedom and portability. It is also lighter in weight.

5.   Over the next 3½ weeks, C.E. seemed to adjust well to his liquid oxygen system. However, one evening he walked to the kitchen for a snack and became increasingly short of breath. Identify 4 possible causes.

As per your instructions, C.E. removed the nasal cannula, tested the flow against his check, and felt no oxygen flowing from the catheter. He lacked the force and volume required to yell for help and was too short of breath to return to the living room to check his oxygen tank. He bent forward with his elbows on the counter top, and struggled to breathe. He became more frightened with each passing second, and his breathing seemed to become increasingly more difficult. A minute later, C.E.'s wife found him and reconnected his oxygen tubing. C.E. sat at the table for 20 minutes before he could walk back to the living room.

6.   Why did C.E. assume the peculiar position at the counter top?

7.   A week later you receive a call from C.E.'s wife. She relates the incident from the previous week and tells you that C.E. "doesn't want her out of his sight." She asks you to come to the house and "...talk some sense into him." What teaching strategies will you use with C.E. and his wife?

8.   C.E.'s wife asks you what her husband can do to help her around the house. She says, "The doctor told him to go home and take it easy. He sits in a chair all day. He won't even get up to get himself a glass of water. I've got a bad hip and this has been very hard on me." How would you address her issue?

The OT instructs the couple about energy saving ways to complete their housework. They both seem satisfied with their new division of labor. In addition, their church women's group has volunteered to help once a week with laundry, vacuuming, and other stressful tasks.

9. C.E. states, "You seem to know what you are talking about so let me ask you something. I wake up with a headache almost every morning. My wife says its because I snore so loud and don't breathe right when I sleep. Do you know anything about that?" After asking several questions you inform C.E. that it sounds like he has obstructive sleep apnea. Explain the connection between obstructive sleep apnea and morning headaches.

10. C.E. seemed impressed by your explanation. He asks if there is anything that can be done for his problem. You inform him that there is a treatment called continuous positive airway pressure (CPAP). What is CPAP and how does it work?

You comment that C.E. sounds like he has a cold. He replies, "Oh, our great-grandchildren were over to visit several days ago and they all had snotty noses. I suspect that I'll get it pretty soon. The problem is, every time I get a cold it goes straight to my lungs."

11. What information would you want to review with C.E. and his wife about the signs and symptoms of infection and when to seek treatment?

12. Why is it important for people with lung disease to seek early intervention for infection?

C.E. learned to manage his emphysema fairly well. His wife had her hip replaced, made a speedy recovery, and was discharged to home. She suddenly died 4 weeks later from a pulmonary embolus. C.E. was panic stricken at her loss. A psychiatric nurse practitioner was requested to work with him.

Case Study 8

Name: _____ Class/Group: _____ Date: _____

Instructions: All questions apply to this case study. Your response should be brief and to the point. Adequate space has been provided for answers. When asked to provide several answers, they should be listed in order of priority or significance. Do not assume information that is not provided. Please print or write legibly.

A.W., a 52-year-old woman disabled from severe emphysema, was walking at a mall when she suddenly grabbed her right side and gasped, "Oh, something just popped." A.W. told her walking companion, "I can't get any air." Her companion yelled for someone to call 911 and helped her to the nearest bench. By the time the rescue unit arrived, A.W. was stuporous and in severe respiratory distress. She was intubated, an IV of LR at KVO was started, and she was transported to the nearest ED.

On arrival to the ED, the physician auscultates muffled heart tones, no breath sounds on the R, and faint sounds on the L. A.W. is stuporous, tachycardic, and cyanotic. The paramedics inform the physician that it was difficult to ventilate A.W. A STAT portable CXR and ABGs are obtained. A.W. has a 70% pneumothorax on the R, and her ABGs on 100% oxygen are pH 7.25, $PaCO_2$ 92 mm Hg, PaO_2 32 mm Hg, HCO_3 27 mEq/L, BE +5 mEq/L, SaO_2 53%.

1. Given the diagnosis of pneumothorax, explain why the paramedic had difficulty ventilating A.W.

2. Interpret A.W.'s ABGs.

3. What is the reason for A.W.'s ABG results?

4. The physician needs to insert a chest tube. What are your responsibilities as the nurse?

5. As the nurse, it is your responsibility to ensure pain control. In A.W.'s case, would you administer pain medication before the chest tube insertion?

6. The ED physician inserts a size 32 chest tube in the 2nd intercostal space, midclavicular line. Many chest tubes are inserted in the 6th intercostal space, midaxillary line. What factor determines where a chest tube is placed?

7. Given the information above, would you expect to observe an air leak when A.W.'s chest drainage system is in place and functioning?

8. Would you expect A.W.'s lung to reexpand immediately after the chest tube insertion and initiation of underwater suction?

9. The clerk tells you A.W.'s husband has just arrived; A.W. will be admitted to the hospital. How would you address this issue with her husband?

10. You approach A.W.'s bedside and ask about what looks like two healed chest tube sites on her L chest. A.W's husband informs you that this is the third time she has had a collapsed lung. He asks if this trend will continue. How would you respond?

11. A.W. recovered and was discharged home 4 days later with a chest tube and Heimlich valve. The physician connected a 1-way (Heimlich) valve between the distal end of the chest tube and a drainage pouch. Discuss the purpose of this device.

A.W. developed several more spontaneous pneumothoraces on the L and eventually had bleomycin instilled over the L lung to induce scarring. She said, "It felt like someone poured kerosene in and threw a lit match in after it. It was the most painful thing I ever went through."

Case Study 9

Name: _____ Class/Group: _____ Date: _____

Instructions: All questions apply to this case study. Your response should be brief and to the point. Adequate space has been provided for answers. When asked to provide several answers, they should be listed in order of priority or significance. Do not assume information that is not provided. Please print or write legibly.

C.K. is a very healthy, active 71-year-old who called his physician with complaints of chills and fever. After taking a history, the doctor instructs C.K. to go to the hospital for admission. He is given a diagnosis of R/O pneumonia. The intern is busy and asks you to complete your routine admission assessment and call her with your findings.

1. Identify the 5 most important things to include in your assessment.

Your assessment findings are as follows: His VS are 154/82, 105, 32, 103°F. You auscultate crackles in the LLL anteriorly and posteriorly, his nailbeds are dusky on fingers and toes, he has cough-productive rust-colored sputum and c/o pain in his left chest when he coughs. C.K. seems to be well-nourished and adequately hydrated. He states that he "got hives" the last time he took penicillin.

2. Which of these assessment findings concern you? State your rationale.

The intern writes the following orders: regular diet; VS with temp q2h; maintenance IV of $D_5\frac{1}{2}$ NS at 125 ml/h; cefuroxime (Zinacef) 1 g IVPB q8h; cefotaxime (Claforan) peak and trough level with 3rd dose; 6 L O_2/nc; titrate to maintain oximeter (SaO_2) >90%; obtain sputum for culture and sensitivity (C&S) x 3; draw blood cultures x 2 sites for temp >102°F; CBC with differential, Chem 7, and urinalysis plus C&S on admission; CXR on admission and in AM.

3. Review the orders and determine what you would do first.

4. Is cefuroxime appropriate for this patient? State your rationale and indicate what action you would take?

5.   Explain the order for the peak and trough level. How is this information used?

6.   Is the intravenous fluid of $D_5 \frac{1}{2}$ NS appropriate for C.K.? State your rationale.

7.   What is the rationale for ordering oxygen to maintain an $SaO_2 > 90\%$?

8.   What is a culture and sensitivity test?

9.   Why would blood cultures be drawn if the patient spikes a fever?

10.   Why are blood cultures drawn from two different sites?

11.   What general information can be obtained from a CXR?

12.   C.K. recovers from his pneumonia and is preparing for discharge. You know that C.K. is at increased risk for contracting community-acquired pulmonary infections. Discuss 4 strategies for prevention.

13.   C.K. confides in you, "You know, my wife died a year ago and I live alone now. I've been thinking...this pneumonia stuff has been a little scary." How will you respond?

Case Study 10

S.M., a 67-year-old woman with severe emphysema, lives with her daughter. Six months ago, S.M. was admitted to the hospital for respiratory failure with severe hypercapnia. She received aggressive treatment with bronchodilators, mucolytics, and steroids. To improve her oxygenation, she underwent a minor surgical procedure for placement of a transtracheal (TT) catheter. She was discharged on bronchodilator and steroid therapy and continued to do well until last evening when she became profoundly short of breath and had to sit in a chair all night. This morning, the admitting nurse interviews S.M. to determine why she came to the pulmonary clinic.

1. What is hypercapnia?

2. S.M. has a TT O_2 catheter at 4 L/min. Describe the catheter and identify its function.

3. Identify 5 complications associated with TT O_2 therapy.

4. There is a possibility that S.M.'s TT catheter is occluded. What should the nurse do before removing the catheter for cleaning?

The nurse cleans the catheter and removes several "mucus balls." She then completes a thorough assessment and notes the following. S.M. remains very anxious after the TT O$_2$ catheter is cleared. Her VS are 112/72, 114, 32, 37.0°C on 4 L/O$_2$ per TT catheter. She is dyspneic and uses accessory muscles of the neck and abdomen for respirations. There are scattered wheezes throughout the R lung fields and LUL, rhonchi over large airways, and breath sounds are absent from 4th intercostal space to the base on L side and greatly reduced on the R. Her skin is thin and friable, with multiple ecchymoses over both arms. She has a moderate amount of hard, dark, guaiac-positive stool.

5. Based on the assessment findings, identify 6 possible problems that S.M. may be experiencing.

6. Given S.M.'s history and your knowledge of pathophysiologic processes, explain the assessment findings.

The CXR reveals LLL pneumonia. S.M. is transported to the hospital and admitted to your intermediate care unit for exacerbation of COPD and pneumonia. The doctor writes the following orders: methylprednisolone (Solu-Medrol) 40 mg IV q8h; erthromycin (Erthrocin) 1g IV q6h; cefuroxine (Zinacef) 2g IV q6h; aerosol treatments using albuterol 2.5 mg (0.5 ml) in 3 ml NS alternating with acetylcysteine (Mucomyst) 5 ml of 10% concentration q4h round the clock; iodinated glycerol 60 mg PO qid; ranitidine (Zantac) 150 mg PO bid.

7. Describe why each of the medications are prescribed for S.M.

8. While you are administering the first dose of medication, S.M. states, "I don't want to be intubated again and placed on that breathing machine. I have lived with my lung disease for 30 years and I'd rather die than live on that machine." What action(s) would you take next? State your rationale.

You arrange a family conference with S.M., her daughter, the physician, and yourself. After some discussion, the physician assures S.M. that medical management will focus on resolving the pneumonia and keeping her comfortable and that her wishes regarding no resuscitation efforts will be respected. The physician details the instructions in the physician orders.

9.   Describe how palliative care differs from curative care.

10. Formulate a list of 8 nursing diagnoses for S.M.

11. Before leaving, the daughter stops you in the hallway and says, "I know that the doctor only gave my mother a 50% chance of survival. I realize how sick she is, but I would like to know if there is anything I can do to better her odds and make her more comfortable." How would you respond?

S.M. was discharged home with a referral for hospice care. Her daughter wrote a "Thank You" note to the nurses on your floor informing you that her mother died peacefully at home 2 weeks later.

Case Study 11

Name: _____ Class/Group: _____ Date: _____

Instructions: All questions apply to this case study. Your response should be brief and to the point. Adequate space has been provided for answers. When asked to provide several answers, they should be listed in order of priority or significance. Do not assume information that is not provided. Please print or write legibly.

The ICU nurse calls to give you the following report: "D.S. is a 56-year-old man with a PMH of chronic bronchitis. He quit smoking 12 years ago and exercises regularly. He went to see his doc c/o increasing exertional dyspnea, and a large mass was found in his R lung. Three days ago he underwent an RML and RLL lobectomy, the pathology report showed adenocarcinoma. He has no neuro deficits and his VS run 120s/70s, 110s, about 34, and he has been running a fever of 100.2°F. His heart tones are clear, he has all his pulses, and has an IV of $D_5 \frac{1}{2}$ NS at 50 ml/h in his R forearm. He has a R midaxillary chest tube to PleurEvac drain, there's no air leak, and it's draining small amounts of serosanguinous fluid. He's complaining of pain at the insertion site but the site looks good, and the dressing is dry and intact. He's on 5 L O_2. He refuses pain medication. He's a real nervous guy and hasn't slept since surgery. He'll be there in about 20 minutes."

1. What additional information would you ask the nurse to provide at this time?

D.S. is transported by wheelchair past the nurses' station to a room at the far end of the hall. You enter his room for the first time to find him sitting on the edge of the bed with his left leg in bed and his right foot on the floor. You introduce yourself, tell him that you are going to be his nurse for the rest of the shift. You note that he keeps rubbing his left hand over his right chest.

2. What issues/problems can you already identify?

3. List 4 things you would do for D.S.

4.   D.S. states, "I have a nephew who rolled his jeep and busted himself up real bad. He got hooked on those drugs, and I don't want any part of them." How would you respond to D.S.'s statement.

5.   Why is D.S. experiencing difficulty using his R arm? Given the type of surgery D.S. underwent, is this expected?

6.   You administer 10 mg morphine ($MgSO_4$) IM and tell D.S. that you will return in 30 minutes; 15 minutes later he turns on his call light. When you enter the room D.S. says, "I think I'm going to throw up." What are the next 3 things you would do?

7.   D.S. stated, "I started to feel sick a couple minutes ago. It just kept getting worse until I knew I was going to throw up." Given this information, what do you think is responsible for the sudden onset of nausea?

8.   Would it be appropriate to give D.S. a second dose of morphine before reporting his reaction to the physician? State your rationale.

9.   D.S.'s pain and nausea are under control an hour later. You remove the chest tube dressing and note that the area around the insertion site looks slightly inflamed, the tissue immediately around the tube looks white, and there is a small amount of purulent drainage. What action would you take next?

The next day the nurse giving you report says that D.S. has been driving her crazy all day long. She tells you that he is fine but has been paranoid and very demanding. You enter D.S.'s room to see how he is doing and to tell him you are going to be his nurse again today. You note that his head bobs up and his mouth opens, like a fish taking in water, every time he inhales. He says, "I just can't (breath) seem to (breath) get enough (breath) air."

10. Identify 6 possible problems that D.S. could have that would account for his behavior?

11. What 3 actions should you take next and give your rationale.

D.S.'s RR is 46; you auscultate slight air movement over the large airways and no breath sounds distal to the 3rd ICS. He's sitting on the side of the bed with his arms hunched up on the overbed table. His gown is in his lap, he is diaphoretic, you note intercostal retractions with inspiration, and all muscles of the upper torso are engaged in respiration.

12. What would you do next?

D.S. is successfully resuscitated and transferred to ICU. The physician returns to your floor and compliments you on your clear thinking and fast action. The nurse who gave you report comes up to you to apologize. She is relatively new and asks you to explain how you know when a patient is in the early and late stages of respiratory difficulty. She states that she wants to learn from her mistakes so she doesn't put another patient through what D.S. experienced.

13. How would you distinguish between early and late stages of respiratory failure?
    <u>Signs of Early Respiratory Failure</u>

    <u>Signs of Late Respiratory Failure</u>

D.S. recovered. His CXR at 5 years showed no recurrence.

Case Study 12

Name: _____ Class/Group: _____ Date: _____

Instructions: All questions apply to this case study. Your response should be brief and to the point. Adequate space has been provided for answers. When asked to provide several answers, they should be listed in order of priority or significance. Do not assume information that is not provided. Please print or write legibly.

G.S., a 36-year-old secretary, was involved in a motor vehicle accident; a car drifted left of center and struck G.S. head on, pinning her behind the steering wheel. She was intubated immediately after extrication and flown to your trauma center. Her injuries were found to be extensive: bilateral flail chest, torn innominate artery, right hemo/pneumothorax, fractured spleen, multiple small liver lacerations, compound fractures of both legs, and probable cardiac contusion. She was taken to the OR where she received 36 units of PRCs, 20 units of platelets, 20 units cryoprecipitate, 12 units FFP, and 18 L of LR. She was admitted to the intensive care unit postop where she developed adult respiratory distress syndrome (ARDS). She has been in ICU for 6 weeks, her ARDS has almost resolved, and she is transferred to your unit. You receive the following report: Neuro: alert and oriented to person and place, she can move both of her arms and wiggle her toes on both feet; CV: heart tones are clear, VS are 138/90, 88, 26, 99.2°F, bilateral radial pulse 3+, foot pulses by Doppler only; Skin: incisions and lacerations have all healed; Respiratory: bilateral chest tubes to water suction with closed drainage, dressing are dry and intact; GI: duodenal feeding tube in place; GU: Foley catheter to down drain.

1. What additional information should you require during this report?

You complete your assessment on G.S. You note shortness of breath, crackles throughout all lung fields posteriorly and in both lower lobes anteriorly, and rhonchi over the large airways.

2. What is the significance of crackles and rhonchi in G.S.'s case?

3. The nurse from the previous shift charted the following statement, "Crackles and rhonchi clear with vigorous coughing." Based on your knowledge of pathophysiology, determine the accuracy of this statement.

4.   It is time to administer 40 mg furosemide (Lasix) IVP. What effect, if any, will Lasix have on G.S.'s breath sounds?

5.   What action should you take before giving the Lasix?

The 0500 laboratory values are as follows: Na 129 mEq/L, K 3.3 mEq/L, Cl 92 mEq/L, HCO_3 26 mEq/L, BUN 37 mg/dl, creatinine 2.0 mg/dl, glucose 128 mg/dl, calcium 7.1 mg/dl, ABGs on 6 L O_2/nc: pH 7.38, $PaCO_2$ 49 mm Hg, PaO_2 82 mm Hg, HCO_3 36 mEq/L, BE +2.2, SaO_2 91%

6.   Keeping in mind that you are about to administer Lasix, which laboratory values concern you and why?

7.   Given the laboratory values listed above, what action would you take before administering the Lasix and why?

The physician prescribes the following: draw STAT Mg level, if below 1.4 mg/dl give $MgSO_4$ 3 g in 100 ml D_5W over 4h; give KCl 40 mEq in 100 ml D_5W IVPB over 4h NOW; and give CaCl 2 g in 100 ml D_5W IVPB over 3h. The laboratory is called to draw a STAT Mg level.

8.   Given that KCl and CaCl are compatible, would you mix them in the same bag of D_5W? State your rationale.

9.   You open G.S.'s medication drawer to draw the Lasix into a syringe. You find one 20 mg ampule. The pharmacist tells you that it will be at least an hour before he can send the drug to you. You realize it is illegal to take medication dispensed by a pharmacist for one patient and use it for another patient. What should you do?

10. While you administer the Lasix and hang the IVPB medication, G.S. says, "This is so weird. A couple times this morning I felt like my heart flipped upside down in my chest but now I feel like there's a bird flopping around in there." What are the first 2 actions you should take next? Give your rationale.

11. G.S.'s pulse is 66 and irregular. Her BP is 92/70 and respirations are 26. She admits to being "a little light-headed" but denies having pain or nausea. Your coworker connects G.S. to the code cart monitor for a "quick look." You are able to distinguish normal P-QRS-T complexes but you also note approximately 22 very wide complexes per minute. The wide complexes come early and are not preceded by a P wave. What do you think has happened to G.S.?

12. What should your next actions be?

13. What are the most likely causes of the abnormal beats?

14. You notice that G.S. looks frightened and is laying stiff as a board. How would you respond to this situation?

G.S.'s PVCs responded well to treatment. Unfortunately one week later, a large fat embolus lodged in G.S.'s lungs. All attempts at resuscitation failed.

Case Study 13

F.P., a 42-year-old male RN, is admitted to the intermediate care floor for exacerbation of asthma that is unresponsive to treatment. His admission weight is 43 kg and his latest VS are 150/88, 126, 32, 102.2°F. You complete a thorough assessment and document the following. F.P. is slightly confused (Glasgow Coma Scale = 14) and very anxious. His temperature is 102.2°F but his skin is cool and clammy. He is tachycardic, dyspneic, and has a slightly productive weak cough. Wheezing is noted throughout all lung fields, and his anterior-posterior diameter is exaggerated. Bowel sounds are hypoactive, and he denies the urge to void.

1. Explain possible reasons for your assessment finding.

You check F.P.'s laboratory values and find the following: WBC 13.5 mm^3, Hgb 17 g/dl, Hct 48%, platelets 280 mm^3, Na 147 mEq/L, K 4.9 mEq/L, Cl 109 mEq/L, CO_2 31 mEq/L, BUN 35 mg/dl, creatinine 2.0 mg/dl, glucose 134 mg/dl.

2. Which of the laboratory values listed above are abnormal?

3. Relate the abnormal laboratory values to F.P.'s condition. What do the laboratory values indicate?

4. F.P.'s attending physician makes rounds on him for the first time. What information is important to convey to the doctor?

The physician prescribes the following: 800 caloric mechanical soft diet; maintenance IV of NS with 30 mEq KCl/L at 125 ml/h; cefuroxime (Zinacef) 1 g IVPB q8h; albuterol 2.5 mg in 3 ml NS q4h; theophylline 260 mg IVPB over 30 minutes then aminophylline 500 mg in 500 ml D_5W to infuse at 0.5 mg/kg/h; prednisone 60 mg PO q8h; morphine sulfate 20 mg IM q3-4h prn for pain; STAT blood culture and sensitivity x 2 sites; sputum C&S; STAT CXR and ECG; acetaminophen (Tylenol) 650 mg PO for temp >102°F.

5. You know the patient has an elevated temperature. After reviewing the orders, what would you do first?

6. You transcribe the orders listed above. Identify the orders that you should question and state your rationale.

7. You initiate the loading dose of aminophylline and leave the room to prepare the maintenance drip. Identify the drip rate required to infuse the ordered dose of 0.7 mg/kg/h for 12 hours, then 0.3 mg/kg/h?

8. List pertinent side effects of theophylline.

You enter F.P.'s room to hang the maintenance drip and find him barely responsive. His respiratory rate is 58, shallow and gasping. He exhibits an asynchronous or paradoxical respiratory pattern, you detect no breath sounds on auscultation, and he is generally cyanotic. His apical pulse is 164.

9. What actions should you take next and why?

The code team responds immediately. F.P. is intubated. The respiratory therapist begins to ventilate F.P. using a bag-valve device when the endotracheal tube (ETT) fills with thick yellow secretions. She calls for endotracheal suction.

10. Explain hyperoxygenation and why it is important to hyperoxygenate before endotracheal suctioning.

11. There are two methods of delivering the hyperoxygenation breaths: the ventilator or the bag-valve device. Discuss which method is the most reliable.

12. When endotracheal suctioning (ETS) is performed, the suction regulator should not be adjusted above the maximum "low" setting. What are the consequences of having the suction regulator adjusted to a medium or high setting?

13. Why are size 14 French catheters routinely used for ETS in adults?

14. You insert the suction catheter until you feel an obstruction, withdraw the catheter 1 cm before applying suction, and begin to withdraw the suction catheter over a 10-second period. A nursing student approaches you and askes why you didn't rotate the suction catheter as you suctioned the patient. How would you respond?

You remove a large amount of thick, yellow secretions from F.P.'s airway and transfer him to the ICU for stabilization and further treatment. The following day he is transferred back to your unit. Because he is to be discharged tomorrow, you are interviewing him about his support systems. He appears to be agitated. Suddenly he says, "You know, I haven't told anyone, but I think I had a near-death experience the other day. I don't think I've gotten over it yet."

15. How are you going to respond?

Case Study 14

P.R., a 31-year-old woman diagnosed with Guillain-Barré, is being cared for at home by home health care nurses because she requires 24-hour/day nursing coverage. She has been intubated and mechanically ventilated for 3 weeks and has shown no signs of improvement in respiratory muscle strength. Her ventilator settings are A/C of 12, V_T 700, FIO_2 .50, PEEP 5. Her VS are 108/64, 118, 12, 100.6°F. She is receiving enteral nutrition by nasal-duodenal tube (2800 calories/24 hours). P.R.'s three children, ages 3, 4, and 6, are staying with her sister.

1. Why is P.R.'s ventilator mode on assist/control?

2. P.R. is receiving lorazepam (Ativan) 1 mg slow IVP q4h to reduce her anxiety. Identify 2 factors that should be considered when choosing Ativan for P.R.

3. Identify 9 nonpharmacologic strategies that you could use to reduce P.R.'s anxiety, increase her comfort, and reduce the need for Ativan. Be creative!

4. You give P.R. a bath and note that her cheeks billow outward each time the ventilator delivers a breath. What could cause this phenomenon?

5. You try repositioning P.R., place a stopcock in the inflation valve, auscultate the lungs, check the length of the tube at the lip (the tube had not moved), and finally insert more air in the cuff before sealing the leak. Over the next 24 hours, the leak becomes worse and the ventilator's low exhaled volume alarm repeatedly sounds. What action should you take?

6. The physician elects to insert a No. 8 Shiley tracheostomy tube with a disposable inner cannula. P.R. becomes increasingly anxious after receiving the news. How would you prepare P.R. and her husband for the tracheostomy?

7. P.R. undergoes the tracheostomy procedure without complications. When you return in the morning and assess the new tracheostomy you note that the trach tape looks tight. You are unable to insert 1 finger between P.R.'s neck and the trach tape. Discuss whether or not this is problematic.

8. What should your next actions be?

9. You note that the tissue surrounding the incision is edematous. As you palpate the area, your fingers sink into the skin and you auscultate a popping sound through your stethoscope. Is this to be expected?

10. Based on your decision in question 9, what action should you take?

11. That afternoon, a powerful storm causes a power failure. What should you do?

12. Within minutes of the power failure, the rescue unit arrives at the door. How did they know you needed assistance?

13. You evaluate P.R.'s activity tolerance and note that she desaturates when turned to her R side. You auscultate tubular breath sounds in the entire R lung posteriorly. Based on your knowledge of pathophysiology, explain the probable cause of the desaturation.

You notify the physician of the change in P.R.'s breath sounds. The paramedic unit transports P.R. to the hospital where she is readmitted for recurring pneumonia.

14. P.R.'s husband arrived shortly after the paramedics transported P.R. to the hospital. He collapses into the nearest chair, tears begin to roll down his cheeks, and he says, "It has been almost a month now. Are you sure she will recover?" How would you respond?

P.R. underwent aggressive antibiotic therapy and was discharged to home 5 days later. P.R. progressed slowly. It took 4 months for her to recover, but recovery was complete.

Case Study 15

Name: _____ Class/Group: _____ Date: _____

Instrutions: All questions apply to this case study. Your response should be brief and to the point. Adequate space has been provided for answers. When asked to provide several answers, they should be listed in order of priority or significance. Do not assume information that is not provided. Please print or write legibly.

D.Z., a 65-year-old man, is admitted to a medical floor for exacerbation of his emphysema (COPD). He has a PMH of HTN, which has been well controlled by enalopril (Vasotec) for the last 6 years. He presents as a thin, poorly nourished man who is experiencing difficulty breathing. He complains of coughing spells that are productive of thick yellow sputum. D.Z. seems irritable and anxious when he tells you that he has been a 2-pack a day smoker for 38 years. He complains that he sleeps poorly and lately feels very tired most of the time. His VS are 162/84, 124, 36, 102°F, SaO_2 88%. His admitting diagnosis is chronic emphysema with an acute exacerbation; etiology to be determined. His admitting orders are as follows: diet as tolerated; out of bed with assistance; O_2 at 2 L/NC; maintenance IV of D_5W at 50 ml/h; sputum C&S x 3; ABGs in AM; CBC, Chem 7, and theophylline level on admission; CXR in AM; prednisone 40 mg PO tid; cefuroxime (Zinacef) 1 g IVPB q8h; theophylline (Theo-Dur) 300 mg PO bid; albuterol aerosolized 2.5 mg (0.5 ml) in 3 ml NS q6h; enalapril (Vasotec) 10 mg PO q AM.

1. Explain the pathophysiology of emphysema.

2. Are D.Z.'s VS and SaO_2 appropriate? If not, explain why.

3. Identify 3 nursing measures that you could try to improve oxygenation.

4. Explain the main purpose of the following classes of drugs: antibiotics, bronchodilators, and corticosteroids.

5. What are the 2 most common side effects of bronchodilators?

6. You deliver D.Z.'s dietary tray and he comments how hungry he is. As you leave the room he is rapidly consuming the mashed potatoes. When you pick up the tray you notice that he hasn't touched anything else. When you question him he states, "I don't understand it. I can be so hungry, but when I start to eat I have trouble breathing and I have to stop." Explain this phenomenon based on your knowledge of the breakdown of carbohydrates (CHO).

7. Identify 3 strategies that might improve his caloric intake.

8. Identify 3 expected outcomes of D.Z.'s treatment.

9. You answer D.Z.'s call light and he asks for a carton of milk. You remind him that milk causes an increased production of thick mucus. He replies, "Yes, but you told me that I had to have lots of protein." How should you respond?

10. You notice a box of dark chocolate on D.Z.'s overbed table. He tells you that he wakes at night and eats 4 to 5 pieces of chocolate. Several of your COPD patients have identified a craving for chocolate in the past. What is the basis for this craving?

11. What would you do to address dietary and nutritional teaching needs with D.Z. and his wife?

12. List 6 educational topics that you need to explore with D.Z.

D.Z.'s wife approaches you in the hallway and says, "I don't know what to do. My husband used to be so active before he retired 6 months ago. Since then he's lost 35 pounds. He is afraid to take a bath and it takes him hours to dress—that's if he dresses at all. He has gone downhill so fast that it scares me. He's afraid to do anything for himself; he wants me within calling distance at all times. I have to keep working. His medical bills are draining all our savings, and I have to be able to support myself when he's gone. You know, sometimes I go to work just to get away from the house and his constant demands. He calls me several times a day asking me to come home, but I can't go home and I don't want to. I just don't know what to do."

13. How would you respond to her?

CHAPTER 3. MUSCULOSKELETAL DISORDERS

Case Study 1

M.B. is a 55-year-old woman presenting to the clinic complaining of episodes of feeling "hot and sweaty" during the day and waking up at night soaked with perspiration. Because her sleep is so disrupted, she is tired all day and is having trouble concentrating at work. She says that the episodes are becoming unbearable and is seeking treatment for them.

1. You suspect she is premenopausal. You obtain her prior medical and surgical history and her current medication regimen. List 3 questions that would be important to ask in exploring the possibility of menopause being related to her symptoms.

2. You are concerned with the possible development of osteoporosis in M.B. List at least 8 questions you would ask to determine her risk for development of osteoporosis.

3. She is not currently taking estrogen replacement therapy. What 3 questions would be important to ask M.B. to determine if there are any contraindications or precautions to this therapy for her?

4. M.B. says that she does have frequent "backaches." Spinal films are ordered. Later you receive a report stating that the films appear normal with no significant findings. What would be an appropriate explanation of these findings?

5.   What would be appropriate supportive measures for M.B. to relieve the noninjury-related low back pain in the absence of fracture?

6.   M.B. reports that she does not like milk or milk products and rarely includes them in her diet. How can M.B. increase her calcium intake at this time?

7.   M.B.'s physician told her that her blood calcium was normal. "If I have enough calcium in my blood, I couldn't have osteoporosis, could I?" she asks you. How will you respond and why?

8.   M.B. says she rarely exercises. What advice should be given concerning exercise?

9.   M.S. states she still is not certain she has a well-balanced diet with sufficient calcium and vitamin D. What would you suggest to her?

Case Study 2

Name: _____ Class/Group: _____ Date: _____

Instructions: All questions apply to this case study. Your response should be brief and to the point. Adequate space has been provided for answers. When asked to provide several answers, they should be listed in order of priority or significance. Do not assume information that is not provided. Please print or write legibly.

J.C. is a 41-year-old man who comes to the ED C/O acute low back pain. He states that he did some heavy lifting yesterday, went to bed with a mild backache, and awoke this morning with terrible back pain. He admits to having had several episodes of similar back pain each year over the last 10 years. In the past, the pain has been treated by diazepam, codeine, and several weeks of bed rest. J.C. has a PMH of duodenal ulcer and takes Prilosec for symptom relief. He is 6 ft tall, weighs 265 lb, and has a prominent "pot belly." The ED admitting clerk calls J.C.'s insurance company to authorize payment for treatment at your facility. J.C.'s HMO has identified him as a consumer of "high cost care" with poor prior outcome. The ED is authorized to perform emergency treatment only and the case manager will make a home visit within 24 hours to devise a treatment plan. The ED physician diagnoses muscular strain of the lower back and orders the following: cyclobenzaprene (Flexeril) 10 mg QID, Feldene 20 mg QD; bed rest for 2 days then gradually increase activity; ice packs to the lower back 30 minutes out of every hour.

You are a case manager (RN) working for Grubabuck HMO and make the initial visit to J.C.'s residence. His wife lets you in and you find J.C. lying on the sofa with his knees flexed and watching videos.

1. What questions would be appropriate to ask J.C. in evaluating the extent of his back pain and injury?

2. What observable characteristic does J.C. have that makes him highly susceptible to low back injury and chronic pain?

3. Why do you think that cyclobenzaprine was prescribed instead of diazepam?

4. What does J.C. need to know concerning Feldene considering his PMH?

You determine that J.C. needs an interdisciplinary approach to treatment and rehabilitation for his chronic back problem. Your goal is to minimize J.C.'s long-term health care costs by rehabilitating his back, helping him reduce his weight to reduce stress on his back, and treating his current injury. You coordinate referrals for J.C. to see four health care experts on your team.

5. You refer J.C. to a physiatrist. What is a physiatrist, and what can a physiatrist do to help J.C.?

6. What expert would work with J.C. to help him lose weight? What are her/his credentials?

7. What kind of expert will work with J.C. using exercise and various treatment modalities to restore his back muscles?

8. What kind of expert will work with J.C. on body mechanics and strengthening him for occupational- and home-related work?

9. A physical therapist teaches J.C. maintenance exercises he can do on his own to promote back health. What 3 common exercises would be included?

Case Study 3

D.M., a 25-year-old man, hops into the ED complaining of right ankle pain. He states that he was playing basketball and stepped on another player's foot, inverting his ankle. You note swelling over the lateral malleolus down to the area of the 4th and 5th metatarsal, and pedal pulses are 3+ bilaterally. His VS are 124/76, 82, 18. He has no allergies and takes no medication. He states he has no prior surgeries or medical problems.

1. When assessing D.M.'s injured ankle, what should be evaluated?

2. What should initial nursing management of the ankle involve that would prevent further swelling and injury to the ankle?

3. You note there is significant swelling over the 4th and 5th metatarsal. How would you further evaluate this finding?

X-rays are negative for fracture and a third degree sprain is diagnosed. The physician orders an ankle splint with elastic wrap and crutches with instructions. The physician instructs D.M. not to bear weight on his ankle for 2 days.

4. Describe the technique for applying an elastic wrap. Give the rationale.

5. When instructing D.M. to use crutches, his weight should rest on what part of his body while the crutch is bearing the weight? Explain why.

6. You are to instruct D.M. on application of cold and heat, activity, and care of the ankle. What would be appropriate instructions in these areas?

7. D.M. is given a prescription for acetominophen/hydrocodone (Lortab) for pain. What instructions concerning this medication should you give him on discharge?

8. Four days later D.M. hobbles into the ED and sheepishly informs you that he "did it again, only this time it was touch football." He states that the pain pills worked so well he thought it would be OK. You detect the odor of beer on his breath. What are you going to do?

9. You remove his sock and find a large hematoma forming on the lateral aspect of the ankle. You inquire about D.M.'s pain perception. He states, "It doesn't feel too bad now but I sure saw stars when it popped." What is the significance of his statement?

Case Study 4

S.P. is admitted to the orthopedic ward. She has fallen at home and has sustained an intracapsular fracture of the hip at the femoral neck. The following history is obtained from her. She is a 75-year-old widow with 3 children living nearby. Her father died of cancer at 62 years of age; mother died of CHF at 79 years of age. Ht 5'3", wt 118 lb. She has a 50 pack/year smoking history and denies alcohol use. She had severe rheumatoid arthritis with UGI bleed in 1993 and CAD with CABG 9 months ago. Since that time she has engaged in "very mild exercises at home." VS are 128/60, 98, 14, 37.2°C. Medications: nizatidine (Axid) 150 mg bid, prednisone (Deltasone) 5 mg PO qd, and methotrexate (Amethopterin) 2.5 mg/weekly.

1.   List 4 risk factors for hip fractures.

2.   Place a check (✓) mark next to each of the responses in #1 that represent S.P.'s risk factors.

S.P. is taken to surgery for a total hip replacement. Because of the intracapsular location of the fracture, the surgeon chooses to perform an arthroplasty rather than internal fixation.

3.   List 4 critical potential postoperative problems for S.P., and explain why you think each is important.

4.   How would you monitor for excessive postoperative blood loss?

5.   There are 2 main goals for maintaining proper alignment of S.P.'s operative leg. What are they, and how are they achieved?

6. Postoperative wound infection is a concern for S.P. Describe what you would do to monitor S.P. for wound infection.

7. Taking S.P's rheumatoid arthritis into consideration, what interventions should be implemented to prevent complications secondary to immobility?

8. What predisposing factor, identified in S.P.'s medical history, places her at risk for infection, bleeding, and anemia?

9. Explain 4 techniques you will teach her to help her protect herself from infection r/t medication-induced immune suppression.

Case Study 5

H.K. is a 26-year-old man who tried to light a cigarette while driving and lost control of his jeep. The jeep flipped and landed on the passenger side. H.K. was transported to the ED with a deformed, edematous R lower leg and a deep puncture wound approximately 5 cm long over the deformity. Blood continues to ooze from the wound.

1. What further assessment should the nurse make of the leg injury and what precautions should she take in making this assessment?

2. What would be the most appropriate method for controlling bleeding at this wound site?

3. What is the best way to immobilize the leg injury before surgery?

H.K. is taken to surgery for internal fixation of the tibia and fibula fractures. He returns with a full leg cast.

4. Describe nursing assessment of a patient with a long leg cast involving trauma and surgery.

5. In assessing H.K.'s cast on the third day postop, you notice a strong foul odor. Drainage on the cast is extending and H.K. is complaining of pain more often and seems considerably more uncomfortable. VS are 123/78, 102, 18, 39°C. What is your analysis of these findings?

H.K. returns to surgery. The wound over H.K.'s fracture site has become necrotic with purulent drainage. The wound is debrided and cultured then a posterior splint is applied. H.K. returns to his room with orders for wet to moist dressing changes. The physician suspects osteomyelitis and orders ampicillin (Unasyn), nafcillin (Unipen), and gentamycin (Gentak).

6. As you continue to assess H.K. over the following days, what evidence will you look for that antibiotics are effectively treating the infection?

7. What should H.K. be taught concerning the care of his cast?

Case Study 6

M.M., a 76-year-old retired schoolteacher, underwent ORIF of his R femur. He has been on bed rest for the first 2 days postoperatively. 0600 VS were 132/84, 80 reg, 18 unlabored, and 37.2°C. He is AA&Ox3 (awake, alert, and oriented). No adventitious heart sounds. Breath sounds are clear but diminished in the bases bilaterally. Bowel sounds are active in all 4 quadrants, and he is taking sips of clear liquids. An IV of $D_5 \frac{1}{2}$ NS is infusing TKO in his L hand and should be saline locked in the AM if he is able to maintain adequate PO fluid intake. His lab work shows Hct 34%, Hgb 11.3 mg/dl, K 4.1 mEq/L, PTT 44 seconds. Pain is controlled with neperidine (Demerol) 25 mg and promethazine (Phenergan) 25 mg IM q3h. He is also taking Nitropatch, heparin 5000 units SQ bid, and docusate sodium.

At 2330 on the second postoperative day, you answer M.M.'s call light and find him lying in bed breathing rapidly and rubbing his R chest. He complains of R-sided chest pain and appears to be restless.

1.   What are you going to do?

He is slightly hypotensive, tachycardic, tachypneic, restless, and slightly confused. The pulse oximeter reads 86%, so you start him on 3-6 L O_2/nc. You identify faint crackles in the posterior bases bilaterally; they were clear this AM.

2.   You contact the physician. What information is important to report?

3.   The physician orders ABGs on room air, continuous pulse oximetry, STAT CXR, and STAT 12-lead ECG. What information will the physician gain from each of the above?

4. Why would the physician order a blood gas on room air as opposed to with supplemental O_2?

The ABGs return as follows: pH 7.55, $PaCO_2$ 24 mm Hg, HCO_3 24 mEq/L, and PaO_2 56 mm Hg at sea level. SaO_2 is 86% on room air. Chest x-ray shows a small R infiltrate. VS are 150/92, 110, 28, 37.2°C.

5. What is your interpretation of the ABGs, and what do you think the physician will order next?

6. The V/Q is performed, and the interpretation reads "strongly suggestive of a pulmonary embolus." What are the most likely sources of the embolus?

7. Based on the latest PTT of 40 seconds, the physician orders a heparin bolus of 5000 units IV followed by an infusion of 1200 units/hour. The PTT 4 hours later is >120 seconds. Based on these results, what action would you take?

8. The next day, the physician's orders read, "Coumadin 2.5 mg, PT in AM, DC heparin." What is wrong with these orders?

9. Thrombolytics, such as streptokinase and urokinase, have been beneficial in the treatment of pulmonary embolus. Why would this medication be contraindicated in M.M.'s case?

10. List 3 priority nursing diagnoses for M.M. related to his present status.

11. Several days later, you hear M.M. requesting his son to bring in a "decent razor" because he is tired of the stubble left by the unit's shaver. How would you address this issue?

Case Study 7

Name: _____ *Class/Group:* _____ *Date:* _____

Instructions: All questions apply to this case study. Your response should be brief and to the point. Adequate space has been provided for answers. When asked to provide several answers, they should be listed in order of priority or significance. Do not assume information that is not provided. Please print or write legibly.

You are working in the ED when a 27-year-old man runs through the door with a blood-soaked towel over his left hand. D.W., a machinist, states he caught his hand in an automatic shear and cut off his left index finger. His coworker has the finger wrapped in a paper towel. You grab a pair of gloves while you direct D.W. to lay on a stretcher where you remove the towel and apply firm pressure to the stump with sterile sponges. A coworker takes his VS and announces 196/122, 144, 22. To distract him, you gather information about his PMH, allergies, and tetanus status. He has a history of depression for which he takes Prozac and is allergic to Darvocet. He has no significant medical history other than depression.

1. What is your first nursing priority in dealing with D.W.'s amputated finger?

2. D.W.'s finger is bleeding profusely. Would you apply a tourniquet to the finger or not, and why?

3. An x-ray of the index finger reveals an amputation of the proximal DIP joint. The fracture has left a jagged protruding bone that can be seen from the distal tip. After controlling the bleeding, what would be the appropriate management?

4. What would be suitable treatment of the amputated appendage?

5. D.W. has not had a tetanus shot in the last 10 years. You have run out of adult TD and you only have pediatric DPT available. Would it be suitable to give the pediatric DPT?

6. What factors influence the success of the reattached digit?

7.   List 3 nursing diagnoses for D.W.

8.   You repeat his VS and record the following: 118/86, 78, 18. Do you find the VS changes to be reassuring or distressing and why?

9.   The OR calls for D.M. Before he leaves you need to start an IV. What type of solution would you hang and why?

10.   Why would it be important to further question D.M. about his allergy to Darvocet?

Case Study 8

B.G. is struck by a vehicle while riding his motorcycle and is transported to your ED by ambulance. He is found to have a fractured mandible and multiple fractures of the R tibia and fibula.

1. When a patient comes in with facial trauma such as B.G.s, what two other injuries should you assume exist until ruled out? Explain.

B.G. is taken to the operating room for intermaxillary fixation (wiring of the jaw) and pinning of the fractured tibia and fibula.

2. B.C. returns from surgery with his jaws wired together. What nursing diagnosis or patient problem statement express your primary concern for B.G. postoperatively?

3. What precautions will you take to ensure a patent airway in B.G. if he begins vomiting while his jaws are wired?

4. If B.G. begins vomiting with his jaws wired, what actions should you take?

B.C. is transferred to a rehabilitation facility for treatment of his leg injury.

5. His jaw remains wired. What instructions should you give him concerning oral care and safety?

6. During his stay at the rehabilitation facility, what nutritional teaching does B.G. need to prepare him for discharge?

B.G. has daily dressing changes, antibiotics, and physical therapy; wound debridement is prn.

7. Two weeks after B.G.'s accident, you enter his room to do his afternoon shift assessment. The shades are drawn, he is sitting in the corner with his face to the wall, and you have been told he refused to go to physical therapy this afternoon. He answers your questions in flat, monosyllabic tones. When you ask him what is wrong, he explodes in anger, even more frustrated because his wired jaw keeps him from being able to talk well. What are you going to do?

8. B.G. tells you, "I got a good look at my leg today when the bandage was off...It looks really ugly. I wanted to throw up." What are you going to say?

B.G. was discharged to home but returned to the rehabilitation facility for physical therapy and continued wound management for 3 months. Several months later you see B.G. at the grocery store. You call his name, he waves and walks toward you. You notice that he walks with a slight limp. He tells you that his leg healed but he has pain in his knee when he walks or hikes any distance.

9. What could be causing pain in B.G.'s R knee (remember that his R foreleg had originally been injured)?

10. You suggest B.G. ask his physician about a prescription for a foot evaluation and orthotics. What are orthotics and what purpose do they serve?

Case Study 9

J.F., a 67-year-old woman, was involved in an auto accident and is life-flighted to your facility. She sustained a ruptured spleen, fractured pelvis, and compound fractures of the L femur. On admission she underwent a splenectomy (5 days ago). Her pelvis was stabilized with an external fixator device 3 days ago, and yesterday her L femur was stabilized using balanced suspension with skeletal traction. She has a Thomas ring with Pearson attachment on her L leg. She has 20 lb of skeletal traction and 5 lb applied to the balanced suspension (her L femur is elevated off the bed at approximately 45 degrees, the foreleg is parallel to the bed and lies in a sling that the nurse adjusts on the frame, and the foot hangs freely). This morning S.G. was transferred to your orthopedic unit for specialized care. You are the nurse assigned to care for J.F. on the night shift.

1. You enter J.F.'s room for the first time. What aspects of the traction would you want to inspect?

2. When inspecting the skeletal pin sites, you note that the skin is reddened for an inch around the pin on both the medial and lateral L leg. What does this finding indicate, and what action would you take?

3. You find J.F.'s body in the lower 75% of the bed, her L upper leg is at an exaggerated angle (>45 degrees), the knot at the end of the bed is caught in the pulley, and the 20-lb weight is dangling just above the floor. What are you going to do?

4. When you lift J.F., you notice that her sheets are wet. Because you have lots of help in the room, you decide to change J.F.'s linen. How would you accomplish this task?

5. J.F. tells you that she feels like she needs to have a bowel movement but it is too painful to sit on the bedpan. How would you respond?

6. J.F. expels a few small, hard, round pieces of stool. What could be done to promote normal elimination?

You ask J.F. if she is ready for her bath, and she responds positively. You let her bathe the parts she can reach and engage her in a conversation as you attend to the rest of her body. While performing peri care you notice that the folds of skin around her peri area are reddened and excoriated.

7. Given that J.F. has been on antibiotics for the last 5 days, what is the likely cause of the problem, and what needs to be done to encourage healing?

8. You ask J.F. what she is doing to exercise while she is confined to bed. She looks surprised and states that she isn't doing anything. What activities can J.F. engage in while on bed rest?

9. You realize that maintaining skin integrity is a challenge in J.F.'s case. What measures will you take to prevent skin breakdown?

10. Although J.F. is recovering nicely, she is becoming increasingly withdrawn. You enter her room and find her crying. She tells you that she is all alone here, that she misses her family terribly. You know that her son is flying into town tomorrow but will only be able to stay a few days. What can be done so that J.F. benefits from her family support system?

Case Study 10

You are working in the ED when M.C., an 82-year-old widow, arrives by ambulance. Because M.C. had not answered her phone since noon yesterday, her daughter went to her home to check on her. She found M.C. lying on the kitchen floor, incontinent of urine and stool, and complaining of pain in her R hip. Her daughter reports a PMH of hypertension, angina, and osteoporosis. M.C. takes propanolol (Inderal), nitropatch, indapamide (Lozol), and Premarin daily. The daughter reports that her mother is normally very alert and lives independently. Upon examination, you see an elderly woman, approximately 100 lb, holding her right thigh. You note shortening of the right leg with external rotation and a large amount of swelling at the proximal thigh and right hip. M.C. is oriented to person only and is confused about place and time. M.C.'s VS are 90/65, 120, 24, 36.4° C; her SaO_2 is 89%. Preliminary diagnosis is fracture of the right hip.

1. In view of M.C. history of hypertension and the fact that she has been without her medications for at least 24 hours, explain her current VS.

2. Based on her history and your initial assessment, what 3 priority interventions should be initiated?

3. M.C.'s daughter states, "Mother is always so clear and alert. I have never seen her act so confused. What's wrong with her?" What are 3 possible causes for M.C.'s disorientation that should be considered and evaluated?

X-ray films confirmed the diagnosis of intertrochanteric femoral fracture. Knowing that M.C. is going to be admitted, you draw admission labs and call for an orthopedic consult.

4. What laboratory and diagnostic studies would be ordered to evaluate M.C.'s condition, and what critical information will each give you?

5. What are the 5 Ps that should be guide the assessment of M.C.'s right leg before and after surgery?

6. In evaluating M.C.'s pulses, you find her posterior tibial pulse and dorsalis pedis pulse to be weaker on her right foot than on her left. What would be a possible cause of this finding?

7. In planning further care for M.C., list 4 potential complications for which M.C. should be monitored.

8. M.C. keeps asking about "Peaches." No one seems to be paying attention. You ask her what she means. She says Peaches is her little dog and she's worried about who is taking care of her. How will you answer?

M.C. is placed in Buck's traction and sent to the orthopedic unit until an open reduction and internal fixation (ORIF) can be scheduled. M.C.'s cardiovascular, pulmonary, and renal status will be closely monitored.

Case Study 11

E.B., a 69-year-old man with insulin-dependent diabetes mellitus (IDDM), is admitted to a large, regional medical center with severe pain in his R foot and lower leg. The foot and lower leg is cool and without pulses (absent by Doppler). Arteriogram demonstrates severe atherosclerosis of the right popliteal artery with complete obstruction of blood flow. Despite attempts at endarterectomy and intravascular urokinase over several days, the foot and lower leg become necrotic. Finally the decision is made to perform an AKA (above the knee amputation) on E.B.'s R leg. E.B. is recently widowed and has a son and daughter who live nearby. In preparation for E.B.s surgery, the surgeons wish to spare as much viable tissue as possible. Hence, an order is written for E.B. to undergo 5 days of hyperbaric therapy for 20 minutes bid.

1. What is the purpose of hyperbaric therapy, and what purpose does it serve in a patient like E.B.?

As you are preparing E.B. for surgery, he is quiet and withdrawn. He follows instructions quietly and slowly without asking questions. His son and daughter are at his bedside and they also are very quiet. Finally, E.B. says, "I don't want to go like your mother did. She lingered on and had so much pain. I don't want them to bring me back."

2. You look at his chart and find no advanced directives. What is your responsibility?

3. What is your assessment of E.B.'s behavior at this time?

4. What are some appropriate nursing interventions and responses to E.B.'s anticipatory grief?

E.B. returns from surgery with the right stump dressed with gauze and an elastic wrap. The dressing is dry and intact, without drainage. He is drowsy with the following VS: 142/80, 96, 14, 36.6°C. He has a maintenance IV of $D_5.9$ NS infusing at 125 ml/h in his right forearm.

5. The surgeon has written to keep E.B.s stump elevated on pillows for 48 hours; after that, have him lay in prone position for 15 minutes qid. In teaching E.B. about his care, how would you explain the rationale for these orders?

6. In reviewing E.B.'s medical history, what factor may affect the condition of E.B.'s stump and ultimate rehabilitation potential?

You have just returned from a 2-day workshop on guidelines for the care of surgical patients with IDDM. You notice that E.B.'s blood glucose has been running between 130 to 180. The sliding scale insulin intervention does not begin until a blood glucose of 200 is reported. You recognize that patients with blood glucoses exceeding 140 suffer from impaired wound healing.

7. Identify 4 interventions that would facilitate timely healing of E.B.s stump.

8. What should the postoperative assessment of E.B.'s stump dressing include?

9. On the evening of the first post-op day, E.B. becomes more awake and begins to complain of pain. He states, "My leg is really hurting, are you sure it's gone?" How would you respond to E.B.'s question?

E.B. will be discharged to his daughter's home with a wheelchair and crutches. He will be evaluated for a prosthesis and begin training when his stump is ready.

10. What instructions should be given E.B.'s daughter concerning safety around the home at this time?

Case Study 12

J.T. has injured his hand at work and is accompanied to the ED by a co-worker. You examine his hand and find a piece of a drill bit sticking out of the skin between the 3rd and 4th knuckle of his left hand. There is another puncture site about an inch below and toward the center of the hand. Bleeding is minimal. J.T. is 41 years old, has no significant medical history, and NKDA (no known drug allergies). He states the accident occurred when a mill at work malfunctioned and knocked his hand onto a rack of drill bits. His last tetanus booster was 3 years ago. It is your job to provide the initial care for J.T.'s injury.

1. You examine J.T.'s hand. What should you include in your initial assessment and why?

You record that J.T.'s fingers are warm with capillary refill <2 seconds. Sensory perception is intact. He is able to flex and extend the distal joints but not the proximal joints of the 3rd and 4th fingers.

2. You notice J.T.'s wedding band and promptly ask him to remove it. Why is this important?

3. J.T. asks you why he can't just pull the bit out and go home. How should you respond to his question?

4. What common diagnostic test will identify fractures and the location of metal fragments in J.T.'s hand?

The drill bit is impaled ½ inch below the surface of the skin, and there are no fractures. Because the hand contains so many blood vessels, nerves, ligaments and tendons, the ED physician decides to consult a surgical hand specialist. The surgeon suspects tendon damage and decides to operate immediately.

5. What do you need to do to prepare J.T. for immediate surgery?

6.   You record that J.T. has had no food since 8:00 PM yesterday and drank "some water" this AM. Based on this information, do you anticipate problems during surgery and why?

7.   Should J.T. be given a tetanus booster before he goes to surgery?

The surgeon repairs two partially severed tendons and wraps the hand in a very large, padded dressing. The distal ½ inch of each digit protrudes from the bulky dressing.

8.   While in the short-stay recovery area, J.T. asks the nurse why his fingers look yellowish-brown. How should she respond to his question?

The surgeon tells J.T. that he had to repair tendons in his 3rd and 4th fingers and instructs J.T. that he is not to work. He gives J.T. prescriptions for an antibiotic and an antiinflammatory agent. He instructs J.T. to make an appointment to see him in the surgery clinic in 2 days.

9.   What instructions should the nurse in the short-stay area discuss with J.T. and his wife give before releasing J.T.?

10. J.T. says, "How in the world is the ice supposed to keep my hand cold with this big bandage on it?" How will the nurse reply?

11. J.T. says, "I'll be able to keep my hand up when I'm awake but what about when I go to sleep?" What suggestion can the nurse make to help J.T. comply with the instructions?

J.T.'s recovery was uncomplicated, and he regained the full use of his hand.

Case Study 13

Dr. C., a 53-year-old nursing professor, comes to your chronic fatigue clinic for evaluation of long-term fatigue, weakness, and pain which have become increasingly disruptive to her life-style. Over the years, she sought medical advice about her fatigue but received vague and often conflicting advice such as "get more exercise," "get more rest," "lost weight," "eat better," "exercise more and lose weight," and "pull yourself together." Despite treatment for "depression," the fatigue remains unrelenting. Nothing seems to help. She confides in you that she is so discouraged and tired of dragging through each day that she has thought of suicide but it violates her belief system.

1.   You ask her to describe her symptoms. What questions will you ask about her fatigue, weakness, and pain?

Dr. C. describes her fatigue as daily, unrelenting, and worse in the evening. The overall fatigue, together with muscular weakness ("feels rubbery") and "nervelike" pain, is aggravated by activity and long days. She experiences nausea when extremely fatigued. She has difficulty negotiating inclines and stairs. Although rest makes her feel better, she feels guilty about "taking the time." She says she rarely attends social events, is having trouble doing her housekeeping and has had to give up doing yardwork. She tells you she worries a great deal about her future and whether she'll be able to work until retirement.

You take a detailed history in preparation for a physical and psychosocial evaluation. At age 17, she developed polio. She described this experience as sudden onset (over a 6-hour period) with fatigue, high fever (104.8°F) with shaking chills, weakness and aching all over. The next day, she dragged her feet, experienced constipation, became anorexic, had chills, indescribable muscle aches, and constant pain. The asymmetrical muscular weakness affected all her extremities, especially her legs. This was followed by over 6 months of hospitalization featuring the Sr. Kenny method of treatment. The moist, hot packs helped relieve the extreme neuromuscular pain. Together with gentle exercise (swimming pool), they helped prevent contractures. "It was that experience that motivated me to become a nurse," she said and smiled. "It has always been a point of pride that I worked so hard and overcame such a vicious disease." Based on her history and your experience with other patients, you suspect her fatigue, weakness and pain are manifestations of post-polio syndrome (PPS).

2.   What comments did she make (above) indicating that her functional status (ability to function on a daily basis) is currently compromised (list 5)?

3. What questions do you need to ask to gain an understanding of her support systems?

4. Dr. C. admitted she is used to "pushing herself even when it hurts." Then she asks if you think an exercise program would be good for her. How would you respond?

5. Dr. C. undergoes some diagnostic tests to confirm the diagnosis of post-polio syndrome. What type of tests might be used for muscle evaluation?

The diagnosis of post-polio syndrome (PPS) as a source of Dr. C.'s fatigue, weakness, and pain is confirmed by the physiatrist. Dr. C. is surprised that she had never heard of PPS and that none of the other physicians had ever suggested it to her. She expresses interest in learning more about her diagnosis.

6. What resources could you refer her to for further information?

7. On a follow-up visit, you work with Dr. C. on ways to adapt her lifestyle to her limitations. List several prosthetic devices that may help control her fatigue, weakness, and pain, and prevent further loss in muscular functioning.

8. What other suggestions could you make to help her adapt to her limitation?

9. On her next visit, Dr. C. tells you she was "shocked" at the idea of thinking of herself as "handicapped." She states, sadly, "I thought I had beat this years ago, but now my old enemy has come back to haunt me." How do you explain her comments?

Although this case featured someone whose poliomyelitis generally affected the lower body, others experience polio over their whole body, even affecting arm movement and breathing. Many individuals with PPS also develop trouble breathing and swallowing, so a history of polio should always be a question asked on geriatric assessments.

CHAPTER 4. GASTROINTESTINAL DISORDERS

Case Study 1

Name: _____ Class/Group: _____ Date: _____

Instructions: All questions apply to this case study. Your response should be brief and to the point. Adequate space has been provided for answers. When asked to provide several answers, they should be listed in order of priority or significance. Do not assume information that is not provided. Please print or write legibly.

The charge nurse on your surgical floor notifies you that your next admission will be H.C., a 70-year-old woman who has an active gastrointestinal (GI) bleed and has just been informed that she has adenocarcinoma of the lung. Her VS are 130/80, 80, 18, 37.2°C. When H.C. arrives on the floor, no family members are present, she has slightly pink coloring, and denies pain although she does appear anxious. Her PMH (past medical history) includes PUD (peptic ulcer disease) with reflux esophagitis, COPD (chronic obstructive pulmonary disease), hypothyroidism, and "fluid retention." PSH (past surgical history) includes TAH (total abdominal hysterectomy) and appendectomy (1965), benign R breast biopsy (1994), and laparoscopic Nissen fundoplication (1994). Her regular medications include nizatidine (Axid) 150 mg bid, $FeSO_4$ 325 mg qd, potassium chloride (K-Dur) 20 mEq bid, hydrochlorothiazide (HCTZ) 15 mg qd, levothyroxine (Synthroid) 0.1 mg qd, salmeterol (Serevent) 2 puffs bid, and theophylline (Slo-Bid) 200 mg PO tid.

H.C.'s admission orders brought up from the ED include the following: admit to GI unit; Dx (diagnosis) of gastric ulcer, adenocarcinoma of the lung, longstanding COPD; VS q4h; NPO (nothing by mouth); IV D_5 NS with 20 mEq KCl/L at 125 ml/h; I&O; CBC with differential; electrolytes, Chem 20, PT/PTT in AM; UA (urinalysis) on admission; O_2 at 4 L/nc prn to keep SaO_2 >92%; fa,ptodome (Pepcid) 20 mg IV at 12h; no NSAIDs, ASA; Guaiac all stools; call MD when husband arrives.

1. Which orders would require some clarification? Why?

You put in a call to the physician for clarification of orders. In the meantime, you proceed with the admission process.

2. What are the major components of the nursing assessment you will perform on H.C.?

Throughout the assessment, H.C. appears to be SOB. Her sentences are getting shorter with pauses for breathing between. You ask H.C. to stand on the bedside scale. As she stands, she suddenly sits back on the bed c/o dizziness and nausea.

3. H.C. had been admitted for a GI bleed. Reviewing the data above, list possible indicators of gastrointestinal hemorrhage.

The physician finally calls to clarify H.C.'s orders: draw STAT H&H, change IV to $D_5 \frac{1}{2}$ NS at 100 ml/h, titrate O_2 to maintain SaO_2 >86%, and give furosemide (Lasix) 10 mg IVP (IV push) if K >3.8 mEq/L. The lab work returns: Hgb 10 g/dl, Hct 30%, K 3.4 mEq/L.

4. Based on these laboratory findings, what are you going to do?

Dr. B. arrives and discusses the options with Mr. and Mrs. C. It was decided to go ahead with partial gastrectomy to remove the ulcer. The pulmonary consultant indicates that H.C.'s adenocarcinoma has metastasized to adjacent tissues to the extent that H.C. is not a candidate for lung resection. Radiation is planned to begin as soon as possible following this GI surgery.

5. What preop care would you expect to give?

6. In view of H.C.'s history, which part of your preop teaching do you think will be most necessary for H.C. and why?

7. H.C. returns to the floor after surgery. She has had a large wedge resection of her stomach with a partial selective vagotomy and a pyloroplasty. She is quite lethargic with stable VS. Her EBL (estimated blood loss) during surgery was minimal (100 ml). She has an NGT in place to intermittent LWS (low wall suction). What should you know about NGT postoperative management? Be sure to include drainage and emergency issues.

8. If H.C.'s NGT is pulled partially out, what is the best action? Why?

9. The second day postop, H.C. still has an NGT and a pulse oximeter. Where might you expect H.C. to have some skin breakdown?

10. How can the nurse best prevent skin breakdown?

H.C. has no postop complications and is discharged to her home with her husband on the 5th POD (postop day).

11. What warning signs would you teach the patient to call her surgeon for?

12. H.C. is preparing for discharge when she turns on her call light. As you enter the room, she says, "I'm leaking." You examine her incision and note that her surgical wound has opened slightly (dehiscence). What action would you take?

After examining H.C., the physician instructs you to dress the wound with a wet-to-moist dressing. You contact the home health nurses for follow-up care for H.C., and she is discharged to home.

13. In addition to dressing changes, what related services might the home health nurses provide for H.C. and her husband?

Three weeks later, H.C. was discharged from home care and started her radiation treatments.

Case Study 2

Name: _____ Class/Group: _____ Date: _____

Instructions: All questions apply to this case study. Your response should be brief and to the point. Adequate space has been provided for answers. When asked to provide several answers, they should be listed in order of priority or significance. Do not assume information that is not provided. Please print or write legibly.

C.E., a 54-year-old woman, is being admitted to your unit with a tentative diagnosis of liver tumor. She has experienced increasing fatigue, anorexia, and a steady weight loss of 18 kg over the last 3 months. Her current weight is 52 kg; she is 5'6" tall. She bruised easily, has mild to moderate jaundice, experiences a "heavy fullness" in the midepigastric area, and c/o a persistent dull ache in the epigastric area that radiates to her back. She describes the pain as constant but not severe and reports that the fullness never goes away, not even when she hasn't eaten for a long time. As an afterthought she adds, "Its strange that I have lost weight and yet my skirts are too tight at the waist." Current VS are 102/60, 84, 28, 38.0°C. The abnormal laboratory results are WBC 12 mm^3, K 3.4 mEq/L, protein 4.8 g/dl, albumin 2.9 g/dl, total bilirubin 2.5 mg/dl, Alk phos 215 U/L, GGT 665 U/L, LDH 225 U/L, AST 130 U/L, ALT 168 U/L, AFP 9.5 mg/ml.

1. Which labs indicate possible liver tumor?

2. Which of the above labs relate(s) to hepatocellular carcinoma?

3. How would you assess C.E. to evaluate her fluid and electrolyte status?

4. What is the significance of assessing abdominal girth? How would you do this?

5. Based on the information above, you would want to complete a respiratory and a neurologic assessment. Why are these 2 systems important?

6. What diagnostic tests might be used to determine if C.E. has a liver tumor?

7.   C.E. is to go for an MRI. What will you do to prepare her for this test?

8.   The radiologist informs the physician that C.E.'s MRI shows many lesions in the R lobe of the liver. The physician comes to the floor to biopsy C.E.'s liver. How will you assist during the biopsy?

9.   What can be done to minimize bleeding from the biopsy?

10.   The oncologist, C.E., and her husband discuss risks and options for treatment. List 4 general types of treatments used for solid tumors.

C.E. decides to have surgery. She has a difficult time waking up after surgery so she is sent to ICU overnight. Her doctor tells you, "We basically opened her up and closed her—the liver was a mass of tumors and the intestines were also heavily involved. The frozen specimens were malignant. The tumor had invaded the major blood vessels so we couldn't resect anything. Her prognosis is less than 6 months."

11.   How will you approach C.E. when you readmit her to the unit later that day?

You are present when C.E. and her husband discuss the surgical findings with the physician. Both C.E. and her husband are stunned—"You couldn't take it out?!!!" Solemnly the surgeon shakes his head and says he is sorry but there is nothing he can do. He turns and leaves the room. You ask if they'd like to be alone for a while and quietly leave.

12.   When you return to care for C.E., you are rebuffed by an angry woman. "Just leave me alone! I don't need your help! What use is all this anyway?!!" How would you interpret C.E.'s response?

Before C.E. leaves the hospital, you introduce C.E. and her husband to the idea of hospice care. Tell them that C.E. will require home health nurses when she goes home but eventually she will deteriorate and may want hospice nurses to support them both. Give them the hospice card and write the name of a contact person on it.

For more information: call 1-412-921-7373 or write to 501 Holiday Drive, Pittsburgh, PA 15220.

Case Study 3

T.H., a 57-year-old stockbroker, has come to the gastroenterologist for treatment of recurrent mild to severe cramping in his abdomen and blood-streaked stool. You are the RN doing his initial work-up. Your findings include a mildly obese (male-pattern obesity) man who demonstrates moderate guarding of his abdomen with both direct and rebound tenderness, especially in the LLQ. His VS are 168/98, 110, 24, 38.0°C, and he is slightly diaphoretic. T.H. reports that he has periodic constipation. He has had previous episodes of abdominal cramping but this time the pain is getting worse. He has NKDA (no known drug allergies.

PMH: T.H. has a "sedentary job with lots of emotional moments," has smoked a pack a day for 30 years, and had "2 or 3 mixed drinks in the evening" until 2 months ago. "I haven't had anything to drink in 60 days." He denies regular exercise—"Just no time." His diet consists mostly of "white bread, meat, potatoes, and ice cream with fruit and nuts over it." Denies hx of cardiac or pulmonary problems and no personal hx of cancer, although his father and older brother died of colon cancer. He takes no "regular" medications and denies the use of any other drugs.

1. Identify 4 general health risk problems T.H. exhibits.

2. Identify a key factor in his family history that may have profound implications for his health and present state of mind?

3. Identify 3 key findings on his physical exam, and indicate their significance.

Based on physical exam and history, the physician diagnoses T.H. as having acute diverticulitis and discusses an outpatient treatment plan with him.

4. What is diverticulitis? What are the consequences of untreated diverticulitis?

5. While the patient is experiencing the severe crampy pain of acute diverticulitis, what nursing interventions would you perform to help him feel more comfortable?

6. What is the rationale for ordering bed rest?

7. What classes of medications would be prescribed for someone hospitalized for acute diverticulitis?

Metronidazole (Flagyl) or clindamycin (Cleocin) are antibiotics that are used in conjunction with a broad-spectrum penicillin, cephalosporin, or aminoglycoside to treat diverticulitis. T.H. is being sent home with prescriptions for Flagyl 500 mg PO q6h and amoxicillin (Augmentin) 500 mg PO q8h.

8. Given his history, what questions *must* you ask T.H. before he takes the initial dose of Flagyl? State your rationale.

9. What is a disulfiram reaction?

10. Aside from warning T.H. about the interactions just described, what instructions should you give him regarding his Flagyl prescription?

11. What information would you want to know before starting T.H. on ampicillin?

12. What are the signs or symptoms of an allergic reaction?

13. What will you do if the patient indicates a history of an allergic reaction to PCN?

14. In order to prevent future episodes of constipation, what dietary changes would you discuss with T.H.?

15. What measures can T.H. take to avoid recurrent acute diverticulitis?

T.H. returns for a check-up 14 days later, all signs and symptoms of diverticulitis gone. He is working on his lifestyle changes and reports he is walking 30 min qd. Only 10% to 25% of patients with diverticulitis require any surgery (usually a colectomy). Those who do often suffer recurrent uncontrollable diverticulitis.

Case Study 4

Name: _____ Class/Group: _____ Date: _____

Instructions: All questions apply to this case study. Your response should be brief and to the point. Adequate space has been provided for answers. When asked to provide several answers, they should be listed in order of priority or significance. Do not assume information that is not provided. Please print or write legibly.

A healthy 14-year-old boy, R.K., is admitted to an outpatient clinic. About 4 hours ago, he had been rollerblading and fell while jumping some obstacles. His left arm was caught under him as he fell. He had some "sharp" pain in the LUQ immediately after the fall. This pain eased off gradually but is coming back now. His mother brought him to the clinic because he fainted every time he tried to stand up. He c/o nausea and has vomited twice. R.K. appears somewhat pale and slightly diaphoretic. He denies being SOB (short of breath) or dizzy when lying down. VS are 104/52 (supine), 92, 24, afebrile.

1. What are R.K.'s key symptoms?

2. What organs lie in the LUQ (left upper quadrant)?

3. What are the nurse's assessment priorities? (list in order of priority).

4. The clinic is not equipped to care for R.K. What should they do next?

5. While the nurses are waiting for the transport unit, what interventions would they initiate?

6. R.K. is sent by ambulance to your ED, which is 5 miles away. You are the RN receiving R.K.. What do you do *first*?

7. R.K. does not have SOB, dizziness, or N/V while lying down. Given the circumstances of the accident, what is the significance of this statement?

8. R.K.'s CT scan reveals a ruptured spleen; he needs immediate surgery. What additional information do you need to obtain before he goes to the OR?

9. What is the greatest danger of a splenic rupture?

10. Before surgery, which labs should be drawn?

R.K. is taken to OR and undergoes an exploratory laparotomy and splenorrhaphy. Estimated blood loss (EBL) is 1600 ml, most of which was infused by means of the Cell Saver.

11. What is a splenorrhaphy, and why should this be done instead of a splenectomy?

12. R.K. is 14 and he heals rapidly. He is discharged on the 5th postop day after having his sutures removed. What factors may have favored his wound healing?

Case Study 5

T.B., a 60-year-old retiree, is admitted to your unit from the ED. Upon arrival you note that he is trembling and nearly doubled-over with severe abdominal pain. T.B. states that he has severe RUQ (right upper quadrant) pain that radiates to his back, and he is more comfortable walking bent forward than lying in bed. He admits to having had several similar bouts of abdominal pain in the last month but "none as bad as this." He feels slightly nauseated but has experienced N/V during previous episodes. T.B. experienced an acute onset after eating fish and chips at a fast food restaurant. His daughter insisted on taking him to the hospital.

Assessment findings are an AA&Ox3 man of medium build who MAEW (moves all extremities well). Moves restlessly and continually, c/o of notable fatigue. Breath sounds clear throughout, anterior and posterior. Heart sounds clear without adventitious sounds, heart rate regular, all pulses 3+ bilat. Bowel sounds audible x 4 quadrants, abdominal guarding noted with exquisite tenderness to light palpation over R side, especially RUQ. Has sharp inspiratory arrest with palpation of the RUQ. Reports light-colored stools x 1 wk. Voids medium amber urine per urinal without difficulty. Skin and sclera slightly jaundiced. Admit VS are 164/100, 132, 26, 37.46, 36°C.

1.   What structures are located in the RUQ of the abdomen?

2.   Which of the above organs are palpable in the RUQ?

Abdominal ultrasound demonstrates several retained stones in the common bile duct. T.B. is admitted to your floor and is scheduled for an open cholecystectomy in the AM.

3.   Given T.B.'s diagnosis, what laboratory values would be important to evaluate?

4.   List 4 preop preparations that need to be done.

5.   T.B. is medicated with meperidine (Demerol) 100 mg IM for pain. He reports that, on a scale of 1 to 10, his pain has decreased from 10 to 4 in 1 hour. Why is Demerol preferred to morphine sulphate? What else could be done for T.B.'s pain?

6.   What data charted in the assessment are consistent with common bile duct obstruction?

7.   At 2330, T.B. spikes a temperature to 38.6°C (tympanic). He is started on a broad spectrum antibiotic: Imipenem/cilastatin (Primaxin) 500 mg IV q6h. What, if anything, needs to be done before the antibiotic is begun?

8.   T.B. undergoes a cholecystectomy. Why is a T-tube drain installed during surgery?

The first day after surgery, the drainage should have a small amount of bloody drainage. This soon changes to dark green (bile-colored) drainage. Initially the T-tube drains approximately 500 ml per day then gradually decreases. The second day postop, you enter T.B.'s room to complete your shift assessment. You note a small amount of bile drainage on his gown and moderate amount on the abdominal dressing. When you remove the tape to change the dressing, you note that T.B.'s skin is blistered and reddened.

9.   In order to protect the blistered area from further damage, you apply a hydrocolloid dressing, such as DuoDERM, HydraPad, Restore, or Ultec to the damaged skin. What are the benefits of this type of dressing?

10. What measures can be taken to prevent healthy tissue around a wound like this from damage or breakdown?

11. T.B. recovers uneventfully and will be discharged with his T-tube still in place. What does he need to know about this drain?

12. What other discharge teaching does he need?

Case Study 6

Name: _____ Class/Group: _____ Date: _____

Instructions: All questions apply to this case study. Your response should be brief and to the point. Adequate space has been provided for answers. When asked to provide several answers, they should be listed in order of priority or significance. Do not assume information that is not provided. Please print or write legibly.

W.T., a 22-year-old white man, presented to the ED with a complaint of "bad" abdominal pain. The generalized abdominal pain started 24 hours ago but seemed to "ease up" after he vomited. Several hours later the pain returned but had shifted to the RLQ and has remained there. The pain is steadily getting worse. W.T. reports marked nausea and "dry heaves," and he has no appetite. He has also had diarrhea for the last day. VS are 124/76, 92, 16, 38.8°C. W.T. works in a bar, has no health insurance, and his history is positive for tobacco ("1½ packs a day"), ETOH ("6-pack of beer a day"), and marijuana ("couple of hits a day"). He is allergic to PCN ("I itched all over").

1. What organs are located in the RLQ?

2. In what order will the ED nurse examine this patient's abdomen?

3. Next, the patient's abdomen is checked for rebound tenderness. How is this done and what does it indicate?

You note no masses and localized rebound tenderness in the RLQ. W.T.'s lab work returns: WBC 15.5 mm^3, Hgb 14.6 g/dl, Hct 43.8%, platelets 280 mm^3; the UA is unremarkable.

4. One of these labs is markedly abnormal and when combined with the physical findings, is usually indicative of a specific diagnosis. Identify the abnormal lab value, the assessment findings, and probable diagnosis.

W.T. is sent to the OR for an open exploratory laparotomy for probable acute appendicitis. He underwent an appendectomy for a purulent but unruptured appendix and is admitted to your unit at 2330. His VS are stable and his orders include: D$_5$½ NS with 20 mEq KCl/L at 100 ml/h; cefoxitin (Mefoxin) 2 g IV q8h x 2 doses; diet as tolerated; up ad lib; meperidine (Demerol) 50 mg IM q4h prn for pain; when tolerating PO fluid, change pain medication to Tylenol #3 1-2 PO q4h prn for pain; droperidol (Inapsine) ¼ to ½ ml IV q6h prn.

5. Which of the above orders need to be clarified before a dose is given? Explain.

6. Just how will you determine the seriousness of W.T.'s allergic reaction to PCN?

7. What type of reaction is considered an allergic reaction?

8. During the morning report you are told that W.T. has had an uneventful night; his VS are stable, and his IV of $D_5\frac{1}{2}$ NS at 100 ml/h is infusing on time. He received his second and final dose of prophylactic cefoxitin and he had no signs of allergic reaction. He will probably be discharged this AM. What questions do you want to ask the night nurse before she leaves?

9. Indeed, W.T. appears stable and discharge orders are written the afternoon after surgery. What key issues need to be addressed in his discharge teaching?

Many inherent individual factors will affect the scope and direction of patient teaching. Consider W.T.'s background; he works in a bar, his history is positive for tobacco, ETOH, and Marijuana. These factors should not be glossed over. To address them would ensure the best chance of a full recovery.

10. Outline patient teaching on pain that would address these issues.

11. There are several additional areas for teaching that are not addressed above. Can you think what they might be?

Case Study 7

While you are working as a nurse on a GI/GU floor, you receive a call from your affiliate outpatient clinic notifying you of a direct admission, ETA (estimated time of arrival) 60 minutes. She gives you the following information: A.G. is an 87-year-old woman with a 3-day history of intermittent abdominal pain, abdominal bloating, and N/Vs. A.G. moved from Italy to join her grandson and his family only 2 months ago and she speaks very little English. All information was obtained through her grandson. PMH: colectomy for colon cancer 6 years ago, ventral hernia repair 2 years ago. No hx of CAD, DM, or pulmonary disease. She takes only ibuprofen occasionally for mild arthritis. Allergies include sulfa drugs and meperidine. A.G.'s tentative diagnosis is small bowel obstruction (SBO) secondary to adhesions. A.G. is being admitted to your floor for diagnostic work-up. Her VS are stable, she has an IV of $D_5 \frac{1}{2}$ NS with 20 mEq KCl at 100 ml/h, and 3 L O_2/nc.

1. Based on the nurse's report, what signs of bowel obstruction did A.G. present?

2. Are there other signs or symptoms that you should observe for while A.G. is in your care?

3. A.G. and her grandson arrive on your unit. You admit A.G. to her room and introduce yourself as her nurse. As her grandson interprets for her, she pats your hand. You know that you need to complete a physical examination and take a history. What will you do first?

4. The grandson, an attorney, tells you elderly Italian women are extremely modest and may not answer questions completely. How might you gather information in this case?

4. What key questions must you ask this patient while you have the use of an interpreter?

5. How would the description of A.G.'s pain differ if she has a small vs. large bowel obstruction?

6. With some difficulty, you insert an NGT into A.G. and connect it to intermittent LWS. How will you check for placement of the NGT?

7. List in order, the structures through which the NGT must pass as it is inserted.

8. What comfort measures are important for A.G. while she has an NGT?

9. You note that A.G.'s NGT has not drained in the last 3 hours. What can you do to facilitate drainage?

10. The NGT suddenly drains 575 ml, then it slows down to about 250 ml/2h. Is this an expected amount?

11. You enter A.G.'s room to initiate your shift assessment. A.G. has been hospitalized 3, days and her abdomen seems to be more distended than yesterday. How would you determine if A.G.'s abdominal distention has changed?

After 3 days of NGT suction, A.G.'s symptoms are unrelieved. She reports continued nausea, crampy, and sometimes very strong abdominal pain; her hand grips are weaker; and she seems to be increasingly lethargic. You look up her latest laboratory values and compare them to the admission data. Her Na has changed from 136 to 132 mEq/L, K has changed from 3.7 to 2.8 mEq/L, Cl from 108 to 97 mEq/L, CO_2 25 to 31 mEq/L, BUN from 19 to 31 mg/dl, creatinine from 1 to 1.4 mg/dl, glucose 126 to 79 mg/dl, albumin from 3.0 to 2.1 g/dl, and protein from 6.8 to 4.9 g/dl.

12. Which lab values are of concern to you? Why?

13. What measures do you anticipate to correct each of the imbalances described in question #12?

In view of A.G.'s continued slow deterioration, the surgeon meets with the patient and her family and they agree to surgery. The surgeon releases an 18-inch section of proximal ileum that has been constricted by adhesions. Several areas looked ischemic, so these were excised, and an end-to-end anastomosis was done. A.G. tolerated the procedure well and recovered rapidly from the anesthesia in the postanesthesia care unit (PACU). Once on the unit, her recovery was slow but steady. A.G. went home in the care of her grandson and his wife on the 7th postop day. Discharge plans included walking several times per day in the house, importance of cough and deep breathing (C&DB) and use of the incentive spirometer (IS) q2h, and observing the wound for signs and symptoms of infection.

Case Study 8

P.M., a 24-year-old house painter, has been too ill to work for the last 3 days when he arrives at your outpatient clinic. He seems an alert but acutely ill young man of average build, with a deep tan over exposed areas of skin. He reports headaches, severe myalgia, a low-grade fever, cough, anorexia, and nausea and vomiting, especially after eating any fatty food. P.M. describes vague abdominal pain that started about the same time as the other problems. PMH: no health problems, nonsmoker, drinks a "few" beers each evening to relax. Assessment: VS are 128/84, 88, 26, 38.1°C; alert and oriented x 3, MAEW (moves all extremities well) except for aching pain in his muscles; very slight scleral jaundice present; heart tones clear and without adventitious sounds; breath sounds clear throughout A&P; abdomen soft and palpable without distinct masses. You note moderate hepatomegaly; liver edge is easily palpated and tender to palpation. P.M. mentions that his urine has been getting darker over the last 2 days.

P.M. is presenting with the key signs of hepatitis. Lab work is sent for identification of his precise problem. Results: Na 140 mEq/L, K 3.9 mEq/L, Cl 102 mEq/L, CO_2 26 mEq/L, BUN 10 mg/dl, creatinine, 1.0 mg/dl, platelets 86 mm^3, direct bilirubin 1.6 mg/dl, total bilirubin 2.3 mg/dl, albumin 3.8 g/dl, total protein 6.2 g/dl, ALT (SGPT) 66 U/L, AST (SGOT) 52 U/L, LDH 205 U/L, ALP 176 U/L, PT 12 s, PTT 32 s, urine urobilinogen 1.6 E U/L, albuminuria 160 mg/dl, bilirubinuria +, +IgM-class anti-HAV.

1. Which key diagnostic tests will determine exactly what type of hepatitis is present?

2. A Chemistry 20 panel was drawn. Which of the labs listed above specifically indicates liver disease?

3. List 8 or more drugs that can cause increased ALT levels.

4. Considering that the basic pathology of hepatitis involves inflammation, degeneration, and regeneration of the hepatocyte, what type of diet will you strongly encourage P.M. to follow?

5. Differentiate between hepatitis A, B, and C on the basis of the mode of transmission and prevention.

6. Name 3 major activities that can be done in a community to prevent the spread of hepatitis (any/all types)?

7. In P.M.'s case, the IgM-class anti-HAV antibody is positive. This indicates that P.M. is infected with hepatitis A and is in the acute or early convalescent period of the disease. Is this disease contagious? What precaution would you take?

8. Pruritus is usually associated with jaundice. What will you do to ease this problem for P.M.?

9. How would you explain to P.M. the likely progression of his disease?

The acute illness runs a 2- to 3-week course with full clinical and laboratory recovery in 9 weeks for hepatitis A, and about 16 weeks for hepatitis B and hepatitis C. The course of recovery may be longer in 10% of patients and some may even become chronic; fulminating hepatitis may develop, causing death in 1% to 3% of patients.

10. P.M. is living at home with his parents and 8 younger siblings. The youngest is a 4-year-old. His parents ask how to prevent the rest of the family from getting hepatitis. What specific instructions will you give? How will you know that these instructions are understood?

11. Given P.M.'s lifestyle, what specific patient teaching points must you emphasize?

12. List 4 critical nursing diagnoses relevant to P.M.'s nursing care.

Case Study 9

Name: _____ Class/Group: _____ Date: _____

Instructions: All questions apply to this case study. Your response should be brief and to the point. Adequate space has been provided for answers. When asked to provide several answers, they should be listed in order of priority or significance. Do not assume information that is not provided. Please print or write legibly.

John Doe #6, an approximately 50-year-old man, is admitted to your floor from the ED. He is lethargic, has a cachectic appearance, does not follow commands consistently, and is mildly combative when aroused. He smells strongly of alcohol and has a notably swollen abdomen and lower extremities. This man was sent to the ED by local police who found him lying unresponsive along a rural road. He was aroused somewhat in the ED. Examination and x-rays are negative for any injury, and he is admitted to your unit for observation. He has no ID and is not awake enough to give any history or to coherently answer questions. Admitting orders are: admit to E3 with R/O hepatic encephalopathy; IV $D_5\frac{1}{2}$ NS with 20 mEq KCl at 75 ml/h; add 1 amp MVI (multivitamins) to each L IVF (IV fluid); Foley catheter to DD (down drain); HOB at 30 to 45 degrees at all times; tap water enemas until clear; abdominal ultrasound in AM; CBC with diff, Chem 20, NH_3 now and in AM; soft restraints prn; vitamin K 10 mg IM qd x 3 doses; thiamine 1 g IM qd; folic acid 5 mg IM qd; pyridoxine 100 mg PO qd; low-protein diet, eat with assistance only; call HO for any sign GI bleed, DTs, or $140 < SBP < 100, DBP < 50, P > 120$.

1.   Which of the above orders must be done by the RN? By the aide? By the clerk?

2.   The lab work drawn in the ED has come back, the blood alcohol level (BAL) is 320 mg/dl and the blood ammonia (NH_3) level is 85 μg/dl. What do these values indicate?

While you are getting John Doe #6 settled, you continue your assessment. Neuro: PERRL, MAE sluggishly, pulling away during assessment, follows commands sporadically. CV: HR regular but tachy without adventitious sounds. All peripheral pulses palpable and 3+ bilat, 3+ pitting edema in lower extremities. IV of $D_5\frac{1}{2}$ NS with 20 mEq KCl/L at 75 ml/h in L forearm. Resp: breath sounds decreased to all lobes, no adventitious sounds audible, patient does not cooperate with cough and deep breathing, on RA (room air) with SaO_2 at 90%. GI: tongue and gums are beefy red and swollen, abdomen enlarged and protuberant, girth is 141 cm (64 in), abdominal skin is taut and slightly tender to palpation. BS x 4 quads. GU: Foley to DD with 75 ml dark amber urine since admission (2 hr). Skin: color pale to torso and LEs (lower extremities), heavily sunburned to UEs (upper extremities) and head. Skin appears thin and dry. Numerous spider angiomas on upper abdomen with several dilated veins across abdomen. VS are 120/60, 104, 32, 37.3°C. Toxicology screen and electrolytes have been drawn.

3. What is the significance of the spider angiomas, dilated abdominal veins, peripheral edema, and distended abdomen?

4. How would you further assess the distended abdomen, and what is the clinical name for your findings?

5. Which of the following nursing diagnoses are appropriate for John Doe #6 based on the assessment given?
    ___ Altered nutrition, less than body requirements.
    ___ Impaired skin integrity.
    ___ Fluid volume excess.
    ___ Fluid volume deficit.
    ___ Altered thought processes.
    ___ Risk for injury.
    ___ Risk for impaired skin integrity.
    ___ Ineffective individual coping related to alcohol abuse.
    ___ Ineffective breathing pattern.

6. What is your concern about John Doe's nutritional status? What are your objective reasons?

7. Why is the low-protein diet ordered? How much protein is reasonable?

8. How might you respond to fellow staff nurses' remarks, "Why are we wasting time with this 'wino.' He isn't worth the time or money. Why don't they let him die?"

9. A nursing diagnoses that is appropriate for John Doe #6 is "Risk for Injury." Consider at least 3 areas of risk injury, and identify actions you will take to ensure his safety.

10. What are the signs and symptoms of delirium tremens (DTs)?

11. Falls are particularly dangerous for a patient in John Doe #6's situation. Why?

12. The aide asks you why the patient has tap water enemas ordered and how many to do "until clear." You reply with the following.

John Doe #6 survives a rocky course of hepatic encephalopathy and near-renal failure. After 27 days, including a week in the Intensive Care Unit, he is discharged to a drug and alcohol rehabilitation facility. He is employed as a longshoreman; fortunately, his insurance covers his month of in-house intense rehabilitation.

Case Study 10

Name: _____ Class/Group: _____ Date: _____

Instructions: All questions apply to this case study. Your response should be brief and to the point. Adequate space has been provided for answers. When asked to provide several answers, they should be listed in order of priority or significance. Do not assume information that is not provided. Please print or write legibly.

J.S., a 57-year-old salesman, has come to his practitioner's office with a moderate amount of chest pain. He says this pain comes and goes and is worst at night, when it wakes him up. He looks haggard, with dark circles under his eyes, "I've got to get more sleep than this."

1. What are some common causes of "chest pain?"

2. What will you ask J.S. to better evaluate his pain?

3. J.S. says the pain has been waking him up for 3 months. What would you want to know about J.S.'s lifestyle?

J.S. indicates that he has tried taking antacids and some other medicine he bought at the drug store just in case these were ulcers but he gets no relief. He tried some sleeping pills but he just woke up groggy with a headache in addition to the chest pain.

4. What tests will be done to help determine the source of the problem?

5. A barium swallow confirms a large sliding esophageal hiatal hernia. J.S. asks, "What is a hiatal hernia, and what do you mean its sliding?" How would you explain this to him?

6. J.S. asks, "Is 'heartburn' always caused by a hiatal hernia?" How would you respond?

7. J.S. would rather try more conservative medical treatment before having surgery. What measures can he try to minimize his pain? List at least 5.

J.S. writes down all your instructions and is determined to conquer his problem without surgery.

8. What meds are most likely to be prescribed for J.S.? What will he need to know about them?

Two months later he reappears at your office, looking even worse than before. "I just can't keep the pain controlled, especially when I'm on the road."

9. After discussion, J.S. agrees on a date to have his hiatal hernia repaired. As he does this, he looks doubtful but desperate. What do you want to ask him right now?

10. J.S. wants to know how the minilaparotomy (minilap) surgery is different from the larger laparotomy surgery. Using a picture you explain the following.

11. J.S. is to have a mini-lap. What preop teaching will he need?

J.S. went to surgery for an NFP by means of a minilap. The surgery was successful and J.S. went home on the second day postop. Two months later he stops back in when he comes in for an appointment with his surgeon. He has had complete relief of his gastric reflux and can sleep flat at night without waking up.

Case Study 11

J.D., with 2 years of sobriety behind him, has been promoted from longshoreman to nightshift foreman in a warehouse. He has new hope and new friends in his AA groups. Unfortunately, his cirrhotic liver has not recovered from 20 years of heavy drinking, and he still has residual effects. During the past 2 days he has had a "bad cough." This morning he coughed up bright red blood (BRB) and came into the ED. His coughing and bleeding have subsided for now. An IV of D_5 NS with 20 KCl/L at 100 ml/h is started and baseline labs are drawn. He is sent to the floor for observation. Shortly after you admit J.D., you hear coughing while passing his room. You enter and see BRB all over his gown and bed. He looks very frightened.

1. What needs to be done at once?

2. What specific tasks must be done?

3. What do you think J.D.'s emotional state is? How would his body respond to this emotion?

4. Recognizing his emotional state, what can you do to intervene?

5. What treatment options exist for esophageal varices? List in the order in which they are most likely to be tried.

6. The gastroenterologist comes to the unit to perform an endoscopic exam. How will you prepare J.D. for this?

7. The gastroenterologist performs the fiberoptic endoscopic examination. Neither cauterization nor sclerotherapy is successful for more than a few minutes and J.D.'s bleeding intensifies. The physician elects to use balloon tamponade to hold pressure on the varices until J.D. can more safely undergo surgery. What key rule will you observe with this tube?

8. What is the major complication of balloon tamponade, and how can you help prevent this?

9. J.D. looks at you and asks, "Am I going to die?" You know that the operative mortality is 5% to 15% in elective cases and 50% in emergency cases. Even the survivors have a curtailed lifespan because of an increased rate of hepatic encephalopathy and liver failure. How would you respond?

10. What is shunt surgery and why is it done?

11. J.D.'s current H/H = 8.6/26. He is to receive 2 units of fresh whole blood and 2 units of albumin (SPA). How will you know if J.D. is having any negative reactions to the transfusion, and what would you do to intervene?

12. How much will you expect the hematocrit to rise after the transfusion of 2 units of whole blood?

13. Whole blood is rarely given today but might in a case of hepatic compromise. Why?

The blood has infused without evidence of reaction, his VS are stable, J.D. talked to the hospital chaplain at length, and then was sent to OR for a portocaval shunt. He will be transferred to ICU afterward for recovery.

Case Study 12

Name: _____ Class/Group: _____ Date: _____

Instructions: All questions apply to this case study. Your response should be brief and to the point. Adequate space has been provided for answers. When asked to provide several answers, they should be listed in order of priority or significance. Do not assume information that is not provided. Please print or write legibly.

C.W., a 36-year-old woman, was admitted several days ago with a diagnosis of recurrent inflammatory bowel disease (IBD) and possible small bowel obstruction (SBO). C.W. is married, and her husband and 11-year-old son are very supportive, but she has no extended family in-state. She had IBD x 15 years and has been on prednisone 40 mg qd for the last 5 years. She is very thin; at 5'2" she weighs 86 lb and has lost 40 lb over the last 10 years. She has an average of 5 to 10 loose stools per day. C.W.'s life has gradually become dominated by her disease (anorexia; lactase deficiency; profound fatigue; frequent nausea and diarrhea; frequent hospitalizations for dehydration; and recurring, crippling abdominal pain that often strikes unexpectedly). The pain is incapacitating and relieved only by a small dose of diazepam (Valium), Pedialyte, and total bed rest. She confides in you that sexual activity is difficult, "It always causes diarrhea, nausea, and lots of pain. It's difficult for both of us." She is so weak she cannot stand without help. You write CBR (complete bed rest) with side rails up on the Kardex.

1. Identify 6 priority problems for C.W.

2. You enter C.W.'s room and note that she has been crying. You ask what's wrong, and she explains that the nurse who admitted her to the hospital the last time said, "Welcome to death row!" C.W. says that she is knowledgeable about her condition, but she still can't seem to shake that "death row" feeling. She was afraid to come to the hospital this time. What can you do to help this woman?

C.W. replies, "Treat me with respect, and as a person, not a disease. Act like I have the right and intelligence to understand my condition. Recognize that I probably know what I'm talking about when I try to refuse a delicious milkshake. When I'm either NPO or nauseated, please don't pop popcorn where I can smell it! It's pure torture!"

3. Considering C.W.'s weakness, chronic diarrhea, and lower-than-desired body weight, what interventions should minimize skin breakdown?

C.W.'s condition deteriorates on the third day postadmission; she experiences intractable abdominal pain and unrelenting nausea and vomiting. C.W. is taken to the OR for probable SBO and is readmitted to your unit from the postanesthesia care Unit (PACU). Thirty-eight inches of her small bowel were found to be severely stenosed with 2 areas of visible perforation. Much of the remaining bowel is severely inflamed and friable. A total of 5 feet of distal ileum and 2 feet of colon have been removed and a temporary ileostomy established. She has a Jackson-Pratt drain to bulb suction in her RLQ and her wound was packed and left open. She has 2 peripheral IVs, an NGT, and a Foley. Her VS are 112/72, 86, 24, 38.2°C (ear).

4. You review the postop orders before the physician leaves the unit. One order reads vitamin A at 25,000 IU/d x 10 days. Why is C.W. to receive vitamin A?

5. You begin a thorough postop assessment of C.W.'s abdomen. What does your assessment include? List in the order that the assessment should be completed.

6. A nursing student enters C.W.'s room and auscultates her abdomen. She looks at you and excitedly announces that she hears good bowel sounds. You take the opportunity to teach her the proper method of auscultating bowel sounds on a patient who has NGT to continuous LWS. How would you correct her error?

The nursing student follows your advice and listens again. She says "You're right, I didn't hear a thing." You tell her that she can impress her classmates while educating them in the correct technique.

7. C.W. is 4 days postop. During the routine dressing change you note a small pool of yellow green drainage in the deepest part of the wound. You realize the physician will want a wound culture. How will you culture C.W.'s wound?

8. You obtain a wound culture, complete the dressing change, obtain a full set of VS and note a temp of 38.1°C, and assess increased tenderness in C.W.'s abdomen. You call to notify the physician and ask for additional orders. What prescriptions do you anticipate?

9.   What information do you need to send to the lab with the wound culture specimen?

10. The physician calls back and asks you to describe C.W.'s wound. What key aspects of the wound should be included?

11. The physician asks you how C.W.'s stoma and drainage look. What should a healthy stoma and usual drainage look like?

12. Will any aspect of C.W.'s history significantly affect the wound healing process? How?

13. With a fairly significant wound infection developing, why is C.W.'s temperature relatively low?

14. The physician tells you that she will be over to examine C.W. As you tell C.W. that her doctor is coming to talk to her, C.W. says that she feels something wet running down her side. You find the some leakage of intestinal drainage onto the skin, what should you do?

You change the ileostomy appliance before the physician arrives. C.W. is evaluated, and it is determined that she should return to surgery for exploratory laparotomy.

Case Study 13

Name: _____ Class/Group: _____ Date: _____

Instructions: All questions apply to this case study. Your response should be brief and to the point. Adequate space has been provided for answers. When asked to provide several answers, they should be listed in order of priority or significance. Do not assume information that is not provided. Please print or write legibly.

C.W., a 36-year-old woman admitted 7 days ago for inflammatory bowel disease (IBD) with small bowel obstruction (SBO). She underwent surgery 3 days postadmission for a colectomy and ileostomy. She developed peritonitis and 4 days later returned to the OR for an exploratory laparotomy. The lap revealed another area of perforated bowel, generalized peritonitis, and a fistula tract to the abdominal surface. Another 12 inches of ileum were resected (total of 7 feet of ileum and 2 feet of colon). The peritoneal cavity was irrigated with NS, and 3 tubes were placed: a Jackson-Pratt drain to bulb suction, a rubber catheter to irrigate the wound bed with NS, and a sump drain to remove the irrigation. The initial JP drain remains in place. A R subclavian triple lumen catheter was inserted.

1. C.W. returns from PACU on your shift. What do you do when her bed is rolled into her room?

2. You pull the covers back to inspect the abdominal dressing and find that the original surgical dressing is saturated with fresh bloody drainage. What should you do?

3. C.W. has a total of 4 tubes in her abdomen as well as an NGT. What information do you want to know about each tube?

4. The sump irrigation fluid bag is nearly empty. You close the roller clamp, thread the IV tubing through the infusion pump, check the irrigation catheter connection site to make sure it is snug, and then discover that the nearly empty liter bag infusing into C.W.'s abdomen is D$_5$W, *not NS*. Does this require any action? If so, give rationale for actions, and explain the overall situation.

The physician arrives on the unit and removes C.W.'s surgical dressing. There is a small "bleeder" at the edge of the incision so the physician calls for a suture and ties off the bleeder. You take the opportunity to ask her about a Demerol PCA pump for C.W., and the physician says she will go write the orders right away.

5. Postop pain will be a problem for C.W. after the anesthesia wears off. How do you plan to address this?

6. Pharmacy delivers C.W.'s first bag of TPN. The physician has written for you to start the TPN at a rate of 60 ml/h and decrease the maintenance IV rate by the same amount. What is the purpose of this order?

7. The physician did not specifically order glucose monitoring but you know that it should be initiated. You plan to conduct a finger stick q2h for the first several hours. What is your rationale?

8. C.W.'s blood glucose increased temporarily but by the next day it dropped to an average of 70 to 80 mg/dl and has remained there for 2 days. Her VS are stable but her abdominal wound shows no signs of healing. She has lost 1 kg over the 3 days. What do these data mean?

You discuss your concerns with C.W.'s physician, and she agrees to request a consult from a registered dietitian. After gathering data and making several calculations, the dietitian made recommendations to the attending physician. The TPN orders were adjusted, C.W. began to slowly gain weight and her wound showed signs of healing. Nutritional problems in clinical populations can be complex and often require special attention.

9. You and a coworker read the following in C.W.'s progress notes: "Wound healing by secondary closure. Formation of granular tissue with epithelialization noted around edges. Have requested dietitian to consult on ongoing basis. Will continue to follow." Your coworker turns to you and asks if you know what that means. How would you explain?

10. Both of you start to discuss what specific digestive difficulties C.W. is likely to face in the future. What problems might C.W. be prone to develop after having so much of her bowel removed?

11. The dietitian consults with C.W. about dietary needs. You attend the session so that you will be able to reinforce the information. What basic information is the dietitian likely to discuss with C.W.?

12. After 3 days of dressing changes, C.W.'s skin is quite irritated, and a small skin tear has appeared where tape was removed. How can you minimize this type of skin breakdown and help this area heal?

13. What specifics of ostomy teaching do you plan to do.

C.W. successfully battled peritonitis. Gradually tubes were removed as she grew stronger with TPN and time. C.W. learned how to change her ostomy appliance and was discharged to home.

Case Study 14

Name: _____   Class/Group: _____   Date: _____

Instructions: All questions apply to this case study. Your response should be brief and to the point. Adequate space has been provided for answers. When asked to provide several answers, they should be listed in order of priority or significance. Do not assume information that is not provided. Please print or write legibly.

B.B., a 72-year-old woman, is admitted from the ED with complaint of constant, severe abdominal and lower back pain x 2 days and SOB over the last 24 hours. "I've had to rest 4 or 5 times gettin' back to the house from the shed—it's gotten real hard to manage all by myself." A niece stopped by and insisted B.B. come into the county hospital ED. B.B. has never received any medical care of any kind. She lives by herself "up the mountain" off of a dirt road in rural Pennsylvania. She is restless, nauseated, and in pain. Everything around her is new and frightening to her. VS are 108/72, 128, 30, 37.9°C (ear), SaO_2 84% on 2 L O_2/nc. B.B. is admitted to your unit at 1900.

1. What possible diagnoses would you suspect with a presentation of severe abdominal pain?

2. The ED nurse giving you report says that B.B.'s admitting diagnosis is R/O pancreatitis. You know that pain control is difficult in patients with pancreatitis. What information will you want to ask the ED nurse before hanging up?

3. B.B. arrives on your unit. As she is getting into bed you notice that her eyes are very wide and she is looking all around. She seems totally overwhelmed in response to the ED nurse's instructions about how to operate the bed. What of the above information may be used to guide the manner in which you approach B.B.?

4. What approach would you use to obtain a psychosocial history and complete your assessment?

You complete an assessment and note the following abnormalities: restless, prefers to sit on side of bed, leaning forward and tightly clutching her handbag. States pain has decreased "some after that lady jabbed me with that needle downstairs." Skin cool, diaphoretic, and pale. Heart rate irregular and tachy. Peripheral pulses weakly palpable x 4 extremities. Resp rapid but unlabored on 2 L O_2/nc, SaO_2 85%, breath sounds absent at the base of the LLL (left lower lobe) posteriorly. Reports marked nausea without emesis. BS hypoactive x 4 quads. Abdomen distended and exquisitely tender throughout to light palpation, guarding noted. Has not voided but states that she has "made less water than usual." Poor skin turgor, dry mucous membranes, mild scleral jaundice.

5. How are you going to assess B.B.'s pain?

B.B.'s admission labs return: Na 148 mEq/L; WBC 17.2 mm^3; amylase 200 U/L; K 4.2 mEq/L; Hgb 12.5 g/dl; Hct 38%; lipase 375 U/L; Cl 114 mEq/L; LDH 160 U/L; HCO$_3$ 98 mEq/L; platelets 306 mm^3; AST 54 U/L; BUN 26 mg/dl; ALT 46 U/L; creatinine 1.0 mg/dl; ALP 96 U/L; glucose 185 mg/dl.

6. Indicate which lab values are important in the diagnosis of pancreatitis.

7. Reviewing the CBC and Chem 7 results, what results are consistent with your observations on her physical exam?

8. B.B. voids 150 ml dark brown urine 2 hours after admission to your unit. What will you do?

9. The physician orders a 500-ml bolus of NS and Foley to down drain. What do these orders mean, and why are they appropriate at this time? What priority assessment must be done when a fluid bolus is given?

You deliver the NS bolus over an hour and insert a Foley catheter. You are surprised that the color of B.B.'s urine is dark amber, instead of the dark brown urine that you saw in the commode. You send a specimen to the lab.

10. The next time you answer B.B.'s call light, she states that her pain is, "Getting bad again." You are puzzled because she is not used to taking narcotics and it has been only 2 hours since her last injection of meperidine (Demerol) 100 mg. What can be done to improve her pain management?

NSAIDs are added to the pain regimen. You administer the first dose and notice that her bedpan is under the covers and it contains the same dark brown fluid that you noted in the commode. You ask B.B. about it and she states, "Aw honey, that's just my chewing tobacco." She spit, the dark fluid lands in the pan.

11. Is there any connection between heavy tobacco use and the effectiveness of medications used for pain control?

12. Based on your discovery, what action would you take?

13. B.B.'s oximeter alarms at 83% saturated, her respiratory rate is 34, and the IV bolus has infused. You auscultate no breath sounds from the scapula down on the L. You percuss B.B.'s lung posteriorly and hear a dull thud up to the scapula on the L and percuss resonant on the R. What is the significance of your findings?

14. What 2 actions would you take next and why?

The physician orders a STAT CXR, which shows a significant pleural effusion developing over the LLL.

15. Based on the diagnosis of pleural effusion, what treatment will the physician likely perform next and what is your responsibility throughout the treatment?

Patients with subdiaphragmatic inflammatory processes frequently present with pneumonia or pleural effusion. Cloudy, yellow fluid (250 ml) was removed. B.B. was placed on broad-spectrum antibiotics until the cultures returned. She was found to have acute pancreatitis and was eventually released to home. As she is wheeled out of the hospital B.B. tells you, "I'll die up on my mountain before I'll come back here." She probably did.

CHAPTER 5. GENITOURINARY DISORDERS

Case Study 1

You are working on a medical unit in an acute care hospital and have been assigned to care for M.Z., an 89-year-old widow. She was admitted after experiencing a sudden onset of R-sided weakness, followed by mental confusion and expressive aphasia. This combination of factors leads to problems with urinary continence. A Foley catheter is placed to facilitate urinary drainage.

1. Insertion of the catheter places M.Z. at risk for a urinary tract infection (UTI). What are the signs and symptoms of UTI?

2. If M.Z. did not have a Foley catheter, how would your list of signs and symptoms be different?

3. M.Z. developed diarrhea. What special instructions are you going to give the nursing assistant assigned to give basic care to M.Z.?

4. The nursing assistant reports that M.Z.'s 8-hour intake is 520 ml, the output is 140 ml. Is this significant? Generate at least 3 possible factors that could account for the difference. Next to each identify which item would be assessed and how.

5. What factors will you teach M.Z. and her daughters about her Foley catheter.

6. You are the nurse assigned to M.Z.'s care. You notice that the nursing assistant emptying the gravity drain is not wearing personal protection devices. You also observe that the spout is contaminated during the process. What issues need to be considered in protecting M.Z.'s safety? Describe your actions in working with the nursing assistant.

7. M.Z. is scheduled for a CXR. You help the transportation technician transfer M.Z. onto a stretcher and notice that he raises the gravity drain to chest level to make sure the tubing is not caught on anything, then lays the bag on its side on top of M.Z.'s legs. The air vent becomes wet with urine. What breach of technique have you witnessed and what is your next responsibility?

8. As you are changing M.Z.'s Foley gravity drain, she says to you, "Honey, I'm just a lot of trouble. I'm not much use to anyone anymore. Why don't you just let me go?" How are you going to respond?

Case Study 2

Name: _____ Class/Group: _____ Date: _____

Instructions: All questions apply to this case study. Your response should be brief and to the point. Adequate space has been provided for answers. When asked to provide several answers, they should be listed in order of priority or significance. Do not assume information that is not provided. Please print or write legibly.

K.B. is a 32-year-old woman who is being admitted to the medical floor for complaints of fatigue and dehydration. While taking your nursing history you discover that she has diabetes and has been insulin-dependent since the age of 8. She has been in chronic renal failure (CRF) and undergoing hemodialysis for the past 3 years. Your initial assessment of K.B. reveals a pale, thin, lethargic woman in no acute distress. Her admitting chemistries are Na 145 mEq/L, K 5.5 mEq/L, Cl 93 mEq/L, HCO_3 27 mEq/L, BUN 40 mg/dl, creatinine 3.0 mg/dl, glucose 238 mg/dl. Her skin is warm and dry to touch with poor skin turgor, and her mucous membranes are dry. Her VS are 140/88, 116, 18, 99.9°F. She tells you she has been nauseated for 2 days so she has not been eating or drinking. She denies vomiting.

1. What aspects of your assessment support her admitting diagnosis of dehydration?

2. Identify 2 possibilities for K.B.'s low-grade fever.

The rest of K.B.'s physical assessment is within normal limits. She tells you she has an AV fistula in her left arm.

3. What is a fistula? Why does K.B. have one?

4. In assessment of an AV fistula, what physical findings would you expect during auscultation and palpation? Why?

Over the next 24 hours, K.B.'s nausea subsides, and she is able to eat normally. Her physician believes she experienced a viral illness because there was no other etiology found for her nausea. While you are in helping her with her AM care she confides in you that she never really understood what "diet I'm supposed to be on anyway."

5. What information would you seek from K.B. now?

6.   Because K.B. is on chronic hemodialysis what are her special nutritional needs?

K.B.'s complete blood count yields the following results: WBC 7.6 mm^3, RBC 3.4 mm^3, Hgb 8.1 g/dl, Hct 24.3%, and platelets 333 mm^3.

7.   Are these values normal? If not what are the abnormalities?

8.   K.B.'s physician notes that she is anemic and this is most likely the cause of her increasing fatigue. Why is K.B. anemic?

The following day K.B. is discharged feeling much better and with a good understanding of her dietary restrictions. Her iron stores have been evaluated and found to be adequate. Her physician has instructed her to continue her same medications before her admission except for the addition of recombinant human erythropoietin 50 units/kg 3 times a week with dialysis.

9.   What information would you tell K.B. about her new medication?

Case Study 3

M.J., a 36-year-old caucasian woman, comes into the homeless shelter clinic where you work as an RN. She says she needs a prescription for birth control pills to help with her "cramps." She says she is from out of state, "between jobs," and tells you her boyfriend threw her out last night. She says she has 2 children who live with her mother "back home" and tells you she's had 3 "miscarriages." Her LMP was "3 to 4 months ago and irregular, but I don't think I'm pregnant." She denies any chronic conditions or current health problems. Her knowledge of family health history is sketchy. You smell cigarette smoke on her clothing and she admits to smoking 2 packs of cigarettes a day. She vehemently denies ETOH and drug use, and says she does not take any prescription or over-the-counter medication. Her hair is dull, her skin is dry and sallow. She appears to be hyperalert and oriented x3, her eyes dart around the room nervously. You watch her eyes as she looks around the room: the pupil sizes appear to respond appropriately to the ambient light and are equal bilaterally. She is 5'6" but she weighs only 106 lb. Although it is a hot and humid day, she is wearing blue jeans and a man's long-sleeved flannel shirt. When she responds to your request to roll up her sleeve so you can take her VS, you notice she's watching your face for any sign of a reaction. Her arm is covered with bruises that range in color from yellow and yellow-green to brown and blue. As you insert the thermometer into her mouth, you make a mental note of several scars and bruises on her face and a recent cut on her lip. Her teeth do not appear to have been cared for in a long time.

1. How would you summarize the above information for the chart?

2. List 3 reasons she may be requesting the oral contraceptives.

3. From the above description, state 3 pieces of information that indicate she is malnourished.

In all clinical settings you encounter individuals who are fearful and suspicious of health care workers as part of "the system." Because of their past experiences, they are hypervigilant to the possibility or perception of harm, insult, or betrayal. This includes victims with a background of domestic or political abuse, prisoners, homeless, illegal aliens, or non-US citizens (particularly if police and health care workers worked together to torture or interrogate), and minority groups. Often there are questions you would like to ask clients, but it is necessary to wait until you have been able to build an atmosphere of trust.

4. List 4 questions you would like to ask someone like M.J., if you knew it wouldn't threaten her.

5. You are very concerned about the possibility of abuse, but want to approach the question gently so you don't frighten her. Instead of asking her directly about her bruises and scars, what other questions could you use that might be less threatening and could lead you to what you need to know?

The family nurse practitioner (FNP) comes in and introduces herself to M.J. She sits eye-to-eye and asks M.J. a few questions about how she has been feeling. She asks M.J. if she ever had a vaginal exam performed in the past and how it made her feel. She explains to M.J. she would like to do a physical and vaginal exam as part of the evaluation. The FNP and you leave the room to give M.J. privacy for changing into the examination gown.

6. Explain why the FNP talked with M.J. first, before having her change into the examination gown.

7. As you present your assessment to her, the FNP tells you that M.J. is not an appropriate candidate for OCs because of her age and her smoking. Explain the rationale behind this statement.

8. The FNP tells you that her goal is to see if M.J. will allow her to test for HIV status, TB, STDs, take an H&H, and let her do a Pap smear. Explain the rationale for each of these tests in the current setting.

As the FNP conducts a general physical examination on M.J., she explains what she is going to do and how it should feel. She also explains the tests she would like to do and why they would be important to M.J. She makes it clear that there is no charge for the tests. During the course of the examination, M.J. admits that she has not eaten a good meal "for longer than she can remember." She also admits that her ex-boyfriend really was her pimp and he beat her when she didn't bring in enough money. She is afraid he is going to come after her and kill her as he threatened. She doesn't know anyone she can trust; her mother "got custody of the kids several years ago while I was on crack and got sent-up for possession" and she won't talk to her. M.J. also alludes to the probability that she will be engaging in prostitution to "pick up a little cash" by saying, "I gotta earn a living the only way I know how." About your offer to teach her about condoms, she says, "It's OK, honey. I've heard it all."

M.J. allows the tests to be taken. To your surprise, the FNP gives her a 1-month paid prescription for OCs and encourages her to come back for the test results, check-up, and prescription renewal. The FNP also gives her a pass for a good meal and directions to the domestic violence shelter for the night. As M.J. goes out the door, she turns to you both and says, "Hey thanks...you've been real nice to me."

9. Why do you think the FNP gave M.J. the OC prescription despite the clear contraindications?

Unfortunately, M.J.s body was found along the interstate 10 days later. She had been sexually molested and bludgeoned to death. No one ever claimed the body, and no one was ever arrested or charged in her death.

Case Study 4

Name: _____ Class/Group: _____ Date: _____

Instructions: All questions apply to this case study. Your response should be brief and to the point. Adequate space has been provided for answers. When asked to provide several answers, they should be listed in order of priority or significance. Do not assume information that is not provided. Please print or write legibly.

You are working on a medical-surgical floor when you assume the care of K.S., a 52-year-old man who is 3 days postoperative from an appendectomy. K.S. was admitted to the hospital with acute R lower quadrant pain, and R/O appendicitis. During surgery it was noted K.S.'s appendix had ruptured and he experienced a brief episode of hypotension. Hemostasis was immediately restored and he has been stable since that time. K.S.'s VS are 106/70, 88, 12, 100.8°F. His most recent laboratory data are Na 144 mEq/L, K 4.8 mEq/L, Cl 100 mEq/L, CO_2 25 mEq/L, BUN 84 mg/dl, creatinine 8.4 mg/dl, glucose 106 mg/dl. Yesterday K.S.'s physician had noted in his progress note that K.S. had acute tubular necrosis.

1.   What is acute tubular necrosis (ATN)?

K.S.'s medications include gentamicin (Garamycin) 80 mg IVPB q8h. MSO_4 1-10 mg IV q4h prn for pain, and acetaminophen (Tylenol) 650 mg q4h prn for fever.

2.   K.S. has 3 potential causes for ATN. What are they?

3.   K.S. informs you he is having incisional pain. What information should you assess before administering his MSO_4 that is ordered?

4. What correlation do rising creatinine (Cr) levels have with the number of functioning nephrons?

5. K.S.'s BUN and Cr are markedly elevated. Do these elevations correlate with his risk of developing chronic renal failure?

6. S.M. calls you into his room and states, "My arm hurts where the IV is." What should you do?

7. You inspect S.M.s's IV site and note the site has no erythema, drainage, or swelling. The IV infuses freely when the dial a flow is wide open. S.M. continues to complain of tenderness at the site. What is another potential cause for his pain, and what are appropriate nursing interventions?

8. What are general nursing priorities for patients in ATN?

Case Study 5

You are working in the ED when M.B., a 72-year-old man, enters with a chief complaint of inability to void. His initial VS are 168/92, 70, 20.

1. Are M.B.'s vital signs appropriate for a man his age? If not, what are the abnormalities and offer possibilities for the abnormality.

While taking your nursing history, you discover he is in general good health and leads an active life. His current medications include finasteride (Proscar) 5 mg daily and vitamin supplements. He reports that he hasn't been able to void in 12 hours and is very uncomfortable. He asks if there is anything you can do to help him.

2. During your initial assessment what finding would you expect in regard to his chief complaint?

3. What are your nursing priorities for this patient?

4. After examining M.B., the ED physician asks you to insert a indwelling urinary catheter. What should you include in M.B.'s teaching regarding the placement of a indwelling urinary catheter?

Insertion of the catheter is usually not painful although, he will feel pressure while the catheter is advanced up the urethra. Once the catheter is in place, he should have a rapid relief of his symptoms, and the catheter will be secured into place.

5.   After 2 attempts at placing the catheter you are frustrated because you are unable to advance the catheter without forcing it. What is your next intervention? Why?

After successful placement of the urinary catheter, M.B. reports he is much more comfortable. M.B. informs you he is scheduled for surgery in the coming week because "the doctor told me the pills were not working." M.B.'s urologist calls with the following orders: admit to urology, condition stable; diet as tolerated; NPO after midnight; consent for transurethral resection of the prostate (TURP).

6.   What general preoperative teaching would you provide for M.B.?

7.   What specific preoperative teaching would you provide regarding a TURP?

8.   What psychosocial issues should be addressed with M.B.?

Case Study 6

You are the nurse in a walk-in clinic. A.P. is being seen this morning for a 2-day history of diffuse but severe abdominal pain. She complains of nausea without vomiting but denies vaginal bleeding or discharge. A.P. claims to have had unprotected sex with several partners, some of whom complain of penile discharge. Her last menstrual period ended 3 days ago. She has no known medication allergies and denies previous medical or psychiatric problems. VS are 108/60, 110, 20, 100.6°F (tympanic).

Physical exam finds her abdomen is very tender. The slightest touch of her abdomen causes her to "jump off the exam table." Bowel sounds are normal in all quadrants. Pelvic exam found purulent material pooled in the vaginal vault, it appeared to be coming from the cervix. A sample of the vaginal drainage was obtained and sent for culture.

1.   What medical interventions can you anticipate?

2.   Based on A.P.'s stated history and the results of the vaginal exam, the physician suspects a *Chlamydia* infection. Formulate a nursing plan for A.P. that can be shared with the community agency for follow-up.

3.   Based on the previous question, identify the potential issues for noncompliance and what other action might encourage successful compliance.

The physician has the option of treating A.P. by one of two different methods. First, the physician could prescribe treatment over a period of 1 week; A.P. would be given the first dose of doxycycline (Monodox) 100 mg PO then would be given a prescription for the same to be taken PO bid x 7 days. Second, the physician could prescribe a one-time dose of azithromycin (Zithromax) 1 g PO which could be administered in the clinic.

4. A one-time dose of azithromycin 1 g PO is ordered for A.P.. Why is this a good choice for her?

5. *Chlamydia* is considered a sexually transmitted disease that has not been mandated to be reported to the Public Health Department (PHD). Why would the PHD wish to see this become a reportable disease?

6. You ask if someone has talked with her about "safe sex." She laughs and tells you there is nothing safe about sex. Undaunted, you ask if she would be willing for you to discuss the use of condoms with her sexual partners. She tells you that she's already careful; if she doesn't know the guy, she uses condoms every time. How are you going to respond?

7. You ask her if she has been tested for HIV. She says, no, she doesn't know anyone with AIDS, and she doesn't do sex with gay men. Now what are you going to say?

8. You ask her if she would like to be HIV tested; it won't cost her anything and no one has to know—it's completely confidential. She agrees to the test and it comes back positive. What is her prognosis?

Case Study 7

S.M. is a 68-year-old man who is being seen at your clinic for routine health maintenance and health promotion. He reports that he has been feeling very well and has no specific complaints except for some trouble "emptying his bladder." He had a CBC and chemistry survey completed 1 week before his visit, and the results are as follows: Na 140 mEq/L, K 4.2 mEq/L, Cl 100 mEq/L, HCO_3 26 mEq/L, BUN 22 mg/dl, creatinine 0.8 mg/dl, glucose 94 mg/dl, RBC 5.2 mm^3, WBC 7.4 mm^3, Hgb 15.2 g/dl, Hct 46%, platelets 348 mm^3. His VS at this visit are 148/88, 82, 16.

1. What can you tell S.M. about his lab work?

While obtaining your nursing history, you discover that there is no family history of cancer or other genitourinary problems. During further questioning you discover that S.M. has had progressive symptoms over the past 6 months, which include the urge to urinate frequently, decreased ability in starting the stream of urine, and decrease in the force of the urinary steam. The health care provider examines S.M. and reports that his prostate is enlarged and gives a tentative diagnosis of benign prostatic hypertrophy (BPH). The health care provider also orders a clean-catch urine and PSA test.

2. S.M. is curious why this condition would affect his urination. What would you teach him?

3. Why were the additional tests of the UA and PSA ordered?

4. What concepts would you include in teaching S.M. to obtain a clean-catch urine specimen for UA?

S.M.'s UA returns with results that are within normal limits (wnl). His PSA is 2.0 ng/mL. The health care provider informs S.M. his blood work was normal. S.M. tells you he still has several questions. What information would you include in answering his following questions?

5. S.M. asks you, "Do I have cancer?"

6. "Will this condition affect my relationship with my wife?" What do you tell him?

7. Before being discharged, the health care provider gives S.M. a prescription for doxazosin (Cardura) with instructions to take 1 mg/d x 7 days, then 2 mg/d x 7 days, and then 4 mg/d thereafter. What type of drug is Cardura, and what are other indications for the use of this drug?

8. What are the most common side effects for this drug class?

9. From a safety standpoint, what information does S.M. need to know about his treatment with Cardura?

Case Study 8

Name: _____ Class/Group: _____ Date: _____

Instructions: All questions apply to this case study. Your response should be brief and to the point. Adequate space has been provided for answers. When asked to provide several answers, they should be listed in order of priority or significance. Do not assume information that is not provided. Please print or write legibly.

It is a hot summer day and you are an afternoon nurse in an ED. S.R., an 18-year-old woman, presents at the ED with severe L flank and abdominal pain, nausea, and vomiting. S.R. looks very tired, her skin is warm to touch, and she is perspiring. She paces about the room doubled-over and is clutching her abdomen. S.R. tells you that the pain started early this morning and has been pretty steady for 6 hours. Her abdomen is soft and without tenderness but her L flank is extremely tender to touch/palpation. She is obviously in a great deal of pain. You place S.R. in one of the exam rooms and take the following VS: 138/88, 90, 20, 99°F. Urinalysis shows hematuria. A flat plate x-ray of the abdomen and an intravenous pyelogram (IVP) confirm the diagnosis of a kidney stone low in the L ureter.

Her mother is in the waiting area and seems to be intoxicated. She is quite noisy, belligerent, and has a strong smell of alcohol. She is obviously upsetting her daughter and is disturbing other patients and their families. The mother is berating you and the other staff members in her loudest voice, "You need to do something, NOW. Don't you know how to do anything?"

1.   What is your first priority and why?

S.R. is seen by a urologist. His plan is to control her pain, prevent infection, and encourage fluids to flush out the stone. She received a dose of intravenous meperidine (Demerol), which eases her pain for the time being. His orders are as follows: discharge to home, encourage fluids, and strain all urine. Prescriptions include oxycodone (Percocet) 1 or 2 tabs PO q3-4h for pain and ciprofloxasin (Cipro) 250 mg PO q12h.

2.   What specific instructions will you give S.R. about her urine, fluid intake, medications, and activity?

3. What factors may impede S.R.'s comprehension of your instructions, and how can you increase her retention of important information?

4. S.R. is quite young to develop a renal calculi. She may need to understand how she can prevent the development of stones in the future. What factors lead to development of the stones.

5. The urologist schedules S.R. for a follow-up visit in 2 days. He informs her that if the stone has not passed by then he will schedule her for extracorporeal shock-wave lithotripsy (ESWL). The physicians' explanation to S.R. is quite technical and confusing to her. In appropriate terminology explain to S.R. the concepts and principles of ESWL.

6. S.R.s' pain has been controlled by the use of IV narcotics. Her mother is still obviously intoxicated. What ramifications might this have on discharging S.R.? Discuss the issues, and generate several possible actions.

7. In view of her mother's condition, you are concerned with sending S.R. home with narcotics. How would you discuss this issues with S.R.?

8. You notice S.R. appears to be embarrassed to discuss her mother with you. How will you respond?

Case Study 9

F.F., a 58-year-old with noninsulin-dependent diabetic mellitus (NIDDM), presents at the ED with severe R flank and abdominal pain, nausea, and vomiting. The abdomen is soft and without tenderness. The right flank is extremely tender to touch and palpation. VS are 142/80, 88, 20, 99.0°F; urinalysis shows hematuria; an IV of .9 NS is started and is to infuse at 125 ml/h. An intravenous pyelogram confirms the diagnosis of a staghorn-type stone in the R renal pelvis. The right kidney looks enlarged. He states that he did not sleep well last night and has not eaten much today. He is obviously very fatigued. His laboratory results are as follows: Na 144 mEq/L; K 4.0 mEq/L; Cl 101 mEq/L; CO_2 26 mEq/L; BUN 30 mg/dl; creatinine 3.6 mg/dl; glucose 260 mg/dl; Uric acid 5.0 mg/dl; Ca 9.0 mg/dl; Phos 2.6 mg/dl; total protein 7.8 g/dl; Albumin 4.0 g/dl; total-bili 0.3 mg/dl, direct-bili 0.1 mg/dl; Chol 200 mg/dl; Alk phos 61 U/L; LDH total 100 U/L; AST (SGOT) 13 U/L; ALT (SGPT) 13 U/L; GGTP 40 U/L; Amylase 98 U/L.

1. F.F. is treated with IV morphine for pain. It is late afternoon before he is admitted to your unit and scheduled for lithotripsy in the morning. What specific priorities do you identify for F.F.?

2. The physician has prescribed gentamicin 80 mg IVPB q8h. You question the physician about giving this large a dose of gentamicin to F.F. You are met with angry and belittling statements. Articulate why you *should* question this specific order for F.F.

3. How should you handle the situation with the physician in order to protect the patient and promote a collegial relationship?

4. Hydronephrosis is a potential complication for F.F. What may be the impact of this problem on his long-term kidney function.

5. Analyze the relationship between creatinine and GFR and predicting kidney function.

6. Later, as you walk past his bed, you notice F.F. crawling off the end of the bed. What are you going to do?

F.F. is going to be admitted. You call the unit nurse to give report. You tell her he's been up all night with pain that has just been relieved by IV morphine. You don't know whether he's going to have lithotripsy or surgery; surgery is unlikely because the stone is so large.

7. You tell F.F. he is going to be admitted and will probably need surgery for his kidney stone. He looks at you, panicked, and says, "I can't do that. I don't have any insurance. This is costing me a wad already." How are you going to respond?

Case Study 10

You are working in the ICU of an acute care hospital and assume the care of E.B., a 78-year-old woman who is 3 days postinferior wall MI. E.B. had been healthy before admission except for a long-standing history of osteoarthritis treated with piroxicam (Feldene) 20 mg daily, and severe long-standing hypertension treated with atenolol (Tenormin) 50 mg daily. She also takes ranitidine (Zantac) to prevent NSAID-induced duodenal ulcers. On presentation to the ED, E.B. had severe hypertension (210/122 mm Hg); therefore, thrombolytics were contraindicated and she was taken directly to the cardiac catheterization lab for acute percutaneous transluminal coronary angioplasty (PTCA). Her angioplasty was successful and she has been pain-free since the PTCA. You are reviewing E.B.'s lab work and note the following values: Na 142 mEq/L, K 4.9 mEq/L, Cl 100 mEq/L, CO_2 26 mEq/L, BUN 28 mg/dl, creatinine 2.2 mg/dl, glucose 158 mg/dl.

1.   What abnormalities are there in E.B.'s lab work?

2.   What are possible causes for these abnormalities?

3.   Describe prerenal, intrarenal, and postrenal causes of acute renal failure (ARF). Given the potential causes of E.B.'s elevated BUN and creatinine, how would they be categorized?

You are given the results of E.B.'s lab work from today. The results are: Na 140 mEq/L, K 5.3 mEq/L, Cl 104 mEq/L, CO_2 24 mEq/L, BUN 68 mg/dl, creatinine 3.0 mg/dl, glucose 104 mg/dl. You have also noted her urine output for the past 8 hours is 160 ml.

4.   Based on these values, what is your next action going to be?

5. Define oliguria and anuria. Which term best describes E.B.'s renal function?

6. In reviewing E.B.'s vital signs you cannot identify any episodes of hypotension since her admission. What might be a possible explanation for her increase in BUN and creatinine?

7. What are your nursing interventions and priorities for a patient in ARF?

8. E.B. has been very quiet. Suddenly she asks you, "Am I going to die?" How will you respond?

9. You talk to her about the possibility of dialysis, which may be a treatment for her. She responds, "You know, I'm 78 years old. I've had a pretty good life and I don't want to be hooked to a machine." What will you say?

Case Study 11

M.Z., an 89-year-old widow, recently experienced a left cerebrovascular accident (CVA). She has R-sided weakness and expressive aphasia with swallowing difficulty. M.Z. has a PMH of L CVA 2.5 year previous, chronic atrial flutter, hypertension, and noninsulin-dependent diabetes (NIDDM). M.Z. has a negative psychiatric history and has lived with her daughter's family in a rural town since her previous stroke. Since admission to an acute care facility 5 days ago, M.Z. has gained some strength, has become oriented to person and place, and is anxious to begin her rehabilitation program. M.Z. is transferred for rehabilitation to your skilled nursing facility with the following orders: hydrochlorothiazide (HydroDiuril) 25 mg PO qd, digoxin (Lanoxin) 0.125 mg PO qd, aspirin (Halfprin) 81 mg PO qd, warfarin (Coumadin) 5 mg PO qd, Tylenol 325 mg q6h prn for pain, zolpidem (Ambien) 5 mg PO hs prn for sleep. Diet: mechanical soft 1800 ADA low Na with ground meat; maintain Foley catheter to down drain; and speech, occupational, and physical therapy to evaluate.

1. What lab orders would you anticipate as a result of this specific list of orders? With each response describe your rationale.

2. Based on the information given, what are the 3 priority nursing diagnoses for M.Z.?

3. At the interdisciplinary care conferences you report that bladder training is progressing and recommend removing the catheter if M.Z.s mobility and communication abilities have progressed sufficiently. The group and M.Z. agree that she is ready. The Foley is removed. Identify 3 problems that M.Z. is at risk of developing following catheter removal. Describe specific nursing interventions for each problem.

4. Two days after the Foley is removed you observe that M.Z.'s urine is cloudy and concentrated and has a strong odor. What are your immediate actions?

5. M.Z. is started on sulfamethoxazole 400 mg/trimethoprim 160 mg (Bactrim DS) 1 tab PO bid x 3 days. However, 2 days later you find M.Z. in the bathroom on the toilet, and she is very upset. There is blood on the floor next to the toilet, and the water is bright red with clots. You help her clean herself, help her into bed, and provide emotional support. Describe your assessment steps. What complications do you anticipate?

6. You complete your assessment and report your findings to the physician. You obtain an order for a straight catheterized specimen for culture and sensitivities. Identify at least 2 causes for M.Z.'s hematuria.

7. M.Z.'s UTI is responding to antibiotics and you want to prepare M.Z. and her daughter for eventual discharge. What specific issues must be considered in the teaching/discharge planning to prevent a recurrence of infection?

8. You talk with M.Z.'s daughter about her understanding of caregiving responsibilities for her mother. What kind of questions are you going to ask to assess whether she is capable of taking on this additional burden?

Case Study 12

Name: _____ Class/Group: _____ Date: _____

Instructions: All questions apply to this case study. Your response should be brief and to the point. Adequate space has been provided for answers. When asked to provide several answers, they should be listed in order of priority or significance. Do not assume information that is not provided. Please print or write legibly.

T.C. is a 30-year-old woman who, 3 weeks ago, underwent a vaginal hysterectomy, right salpingo-oophorectomy for abdominal pain, and endometriosis. Postoperatively she experienced an intraabdominal hemorrhage and her Hct dropped from 40.5% to 21%. She was transfused with 3 units of PRCs. Following discharge she continued to have abdominal pain, chills, and fever and was subsequently readmitted twice: once for treatment of postop infection and the second time for evacuation of pelvic hematoma. Despite treatment, T.C. continued to have abdominal pain, chills, fever, and N/V.

T.C. has now been admitted to your unit following an exploratory laparotomy. V.S. 130/70, 94, 16, 37.6°F (tympanic). She is easily aroused and oriented to place and person. She dozes between verbal requests. She has a low-midline abdominal dressing that is dry and intact and a Jackson-Pratt (JP) drain that is fully compressed and contains a scant amount of bright red blood. Her Foley to down drain has clear yellow urine. She has an IV of 1000 ml D_5.2 NS infusing at 100 ml/h in her L forearm, with no swelling or redness. T.C. is receiving IV morphine sulfate for pain control through a patient-controlled analgesia pump (PCA). The settings are: dose 2 mg, lock-out interval 15 min, 4 hour maximum of 30 mg. When aroused, she states that her pain is an 8 on a 1 to 10 scale. She also has 2 L O_2/nc, and her SaO_2 by pulse oximeter is 93%.

1. During your assessment you note that T.C.s' respiratory rate is 16 and shallow. Articulate your plan for a more complete assessment of T.C.s' condition. Include factors to be considered, the supporting rationale, and your nursing actions.

The unit is very busy when T.C. is returned from the postanesthesia care unit (PACU). Staffing is minimal. You are concerned about monitoring T.C. carefully enough. Your present patient load is 6, 2 patients are newly postop, and 1 is getting ready for discharge. You have a nursing assistant that you share with another R.N. You are most concerned with T.C.s' respiratory status and the possibility that she may, in her drowsy state, self-administer a dose of narcotic that would further reduce her respiratory status.

2. Formulate a plan, given the resources mentioned above.

3. Pain control using the PCA can be very tricky. Throughout the first post-op day it has been difficult to juggle T.C.'s need for pain medication and depression of her respiratory status. Discuss the concepts of controlling pain with IV narcotics and factors that may be adjusted to better control her pain.

4. T.C. is beginning to withdraw from conversations with you and the other staff, she sleeps most of the day, and is not eating. At times she is tearful and is irritable with her husband. You believe that she is showing signs of depression. What actions should you take to help her?

5. T.C. and her husband are talking one evening and you overhear that they are very dissatisfied with the care provided by the physician. They believe that he has mismanaged T.C.'s care. They are discussing getting an attorney. They ask you what you think. What do you do?

You realize threats of legal action are based on many issues. Anger and disappointment are among the most common. You sit down to communicate to them that you are willing to listen.

6. You state, "Legal action won't fix how you're feeling or what you need *now*. Tell me what's going on with you. Maybe I can help." What would be the benefit of taking this approach?

7. Mr. C. says, "No one is telling us anything. My wife came in here for a simple hysterectomy, she ends up with 4 surgeries, she still has pain, and she's worse off than when she started. *Somebody* has screwed up big time. Then they have the nerve to send me a bill. This morning they demanded $185,000. I'm not paying a dime until she gets better." How are you going to respond?

CHAPTER 6. NEUROLOGIC DISORDERS

Case Study 1

M.E. is a 62-year-old woman who has a 5-year history of progressive forgetfulness. She is no longer able to care for herself, has becomes increasingly depressed and paranoid, and recently started a fire in the kitchen. After extensive neurologic evaluation, M.E. was diagnosed as having Alzheimer's disease. Her husband and children have come to your extended fare facility's (ECF) Alzheimers Unit for information about this disease and to discuss the possibility of placement for M.E. You reassure the family that you have experience dealing with questions and concerns that most people in their situation have.

1. How would you explain Alzheimer's disease to the family?

2. The husband asks, "How did she get Alzheimer's? We don't know anyone else who has it." How would you respond?

3. After asking the family to describe M.E.'s behavior, you determine that she is in stage 2 of Alzheimers' three stages. Describe common signs and symptoms for each stage of the disease.

4.   The daughter expresses frustration at the number of tests M.E. had to undergo and the length of time it took for someone to diagnosis M.E.'s problem. What tests are likely to be performed and how is Alzheimer's disease diagnosed?

The husband states, "How are you going to take care of her? She wanders around all night long. She can't find her way to the bathroom in a house she's lived in for 43 years. She can't be trusted to be alone any more; she almost burnt the house down. We're all exhausted; there are 3 of us and we can't keep up with her." You acknowledge how exhausted they must be from trying to keep her safe. You tell the family that there is no known treatment and that Alzheimer's units have been created to provide a structured, safe environment for each person.

5.   Describe the Alzheimer's-related nursing interventions related to each of the following nursing diagnoses: self-care deficits, sleep pattern disturbance, impaired verbal communication, impaired cognitive function, risk for injury.

6.   M.E.'s son asks why different medications might be prescribed for M.E. How would you describe the purpose of antiseizure, antipsychotic, antidepressive, or sedative medications for a patient like M.E.?

You try to comfort the family by telling them that the problems they are experiencing are very common. You explain that family support is a major focus of your program.

7.   List 4 ways that M.E.'s family might receive the support they need.

Note: Alzheimer's disease support groups:

Alzheimer's Disease and Related Disorders Association
919 North Michigan Ave., Suite 1000
Chicago, IL 60611
1-800-272-3900

American Association of Retired Persons
Fulfillment Services
601 E. St., N.W.
Washington DC 20049
1-202-434-2534

Case Study 2

Name: _____ Class/Group: _____ Date: _____

Instructions: All questions apply to this case study. Your response should be brief and to the point. Adequate space has been provided for answers. When asked to provide several answers, they should be listed in order of priority or significance. Do not assume information that is not provided. Please print or write legibly.

D.S. is a 74-year-old retired social worker who has been on your floor for several days receiving qod plasmapheresis for myasthenia gravis (MG). She has a PMH of NIDDM for 3 years and low back pain secondary to spinal stenosis. She received 2 steroid injections into her spine for pain 2 to 3 weeks before her admission, which was followed by progressive, symmetric, weakness in her lower extremities proximal > distal, R foot numbness, poor eye-hand coordination, and significant hand weakness. On admission, D.S. was unable to bear any weight or take fluids through a straw. There have been periods of exacerbation and remission since admission.

1. You are visiting with D.S.'s grandson who tells you he is just starting medical school and he would like to know more about MG so he can discuss it with his grandmother. What do you tell him?

2. He asks you to explain how plasmapheresis works. How would you explain this treatment?

3. He asks what drugs are used to treat MG. You explain that although neostigmine (Prostigmin) and pyridostigmine (Mestinon) are often used in combination, drug regimens and doses are highly individualized. Identify the appropriate drug classification for and explain the action of these two drugs to D.S.'s grandson.

4.   D.S. told her grandson that after taking her morning medications she often experienced nausea, heartburn, slight shortness of breath, sweating, and felt her heart beating rapidly. What can you tell him about this?

5.   Describe a myasthenic crisis.

6.   List 6 nursing diagnoses that would be appropriate for D.S.

7.   List 5 factors that could predispose D.S. to an exacerbation of her illness.

8. D.S. asks you what the doctors meant when they were talking about some kind of a challenge test. You realize they must have been discussing the possibility of performing an edrophonium (Tensilon) challenge. What is a Tensilon challenge and what information will it yield?

9. D.S.'s grandson wants to know when she'll be able to go home. How do you respond?

10. What supportive measures can you suggest to D.S.'s grandson that he can undertake or arrange on behalf of his grandmother?

Before D.S.'s grandson leaves, you give him the following address:
   Myasthenia Gravis Foundation
   222 S. Riverside Plaza Suite 1540
   Chicago, IL 60606
   1-800-541-5454

Case Study 3

J.G. is a 34-year-old PI GI woman who underwent an emergency cesarean delivery after a prolonged labor, during which she exhibited a sudden change in neurologic functioning and started seizing. Since that time, she has experienced 3 tonic-clonic (grand mal) seizures, diagnosed as having a basal ganglion hematoma with infarct, and was started on phenytoin. Postdelivery, J.G. demonstrated dyskinesia, resulting in frequent falls with ambulation. When the seizure disorder appeared to be under control, she was transferred to a rehabilitation facility for evaluation, and 2 weeks of intensive physical therapy. She is now home, where she is doing quite well but still has occasional falls and is receiving physical therapy 3 times a week in her home. She remains on phenytoin and has had no seizures since her release from the rehabilitation facility. As case manager for J.G.'s HMO, you visit her and her family at home for evaluation of long-term, follow-up care.

1. A seizure is not a disease in itself but a symptom of a disease. What is the term for chronically recurring seizures?

2. Does J.G. have epilepsy?

3. The 3 main phases of a seizure are the preictal, ictal, and postictal. Differentiate between the 3 phases, and list clinical symptoms you may observe when a patient is having a seizure.

4. What is the pathophysiology of a seizure?

5. J.G. had grand mal, or tonic-clonic, seizures. Describe this type of seizure. List 5 other types of seizures.

6. Some patients know they are about to have a seizure. What is this preseizure warning called, and what form does it take?

7. Besides the brain injury, what are some other possible conditions that could be contributing to J.G's lowered seizure threshold?

8. List 5 classifications of antiseizure medications.

9. J.G.'s husband comes to visit and asks you what he should do if she has a seizure at home. What would do you tell him?

10. Her husband states that he is afraid for J.G. to take care of the baby. What would you say to him?

11. J.G.'s husband tells you that his wife is not good at remembering to take medication. What are some strategies that you should review with J.G. and her husband to increase the likelihood of compliance?

12. J.G. asks, "If I get my blood level under control will it stay at the same level as long as I take my medicine?" How would you answer her question?

13. J.G.'s husband asks if the drugs could harm his wife in any way. What general information would you give them about anticonvulsants?

14. J.G.'s husband says, "I was watching 'Emergency' last night and they showed this guy who just kept on having a seizure. That doctor had to give him lots of medicine before he came out of it. What is that called?" How would you explain status epilepticus, and why is it a medical emergency?

Case Study 4

You have been asked to see D.V. in the Neurologic Clinic on referral from his internist, who thinks his patient is having symptoms of multiple sclerosis (MS). He is a 20-year-old man who has experienced increasing urinary frequency and urgency over the past 2 months. Because his female partner was treated for a sexually transmitted disease, D.V. also underwent treatment, but the symptoms did not resolve. D.V. has also recently had 2 brief episodes of eye "fuzziness" associated with diplopia and brightness. He has noticed ascending numbness and weakness of the R arm with inability to hold objects over the past few days. Now he reports rapid progression of weakness in his legs.

1. MS is an inflammatory disorder of the nervous system causing scattered, patchy demyelinization of the CNS. What does myelin do? What is demyelinization?

2. MS is characterized by remissions and exacerbations. What happens to the myelin during each of these phases?

3. Isn't D.V. too young to get MS? What is the etiology?

4. What assessment data from the case study caused the physician to suspect a possible diagnosis of MS?

Diagnostic tests are often done to rule out other disorders with similar symptoms. A diagnosis will be made when other disorders have been ruled out, when the patient has 2 or more exacerbations, there is slow, steady progression, and/or the patient has 2 or more areas of demyelinization or plaque formation.

5. What are 4 common diagnostic tests you can begin to teach D.V. about?

6. D.V. asks you, "If this turns out to be MS, what is the treatment?"

7. As part of your teaching plan you want D.V. to be aware of situations or factors that are known to cause an exacerbation of symptoms. List four.

8. The National Multiple Sclerosis Society, 733 3rd Ave., 6th Floor, New York, NY 10017-3288 (1-800-344-4867), is a great resource for D.V. What are some resources available in the community that D.V. may need referrals to?

D.V. confides in you that he tried to commit suicide at the age of 14 when his parents got a divorce. He tells you that he knows his girlfriend hasn't been faithful but he is afraid of living alone. He admits that she occasionally hits him, but he's afraid if he tells her about his M.S. diagnosis she'll leave him for good. You recall seeing yellowish bruises on his arms when you took his admission blood pressure.

9. What are you going to do with this information?

10. In view of his personal history and current diagnosis, what two critical psychosocial issues are you going to monitor for in his follow-up visits?

D.V. took advantage of his time with the psychiatric nurse specialist, joined a local MS support group, and told his girlfriend to move out. He later married a woman from the support group.

Case Study 5

S.B. is a 28-year-old married woman with a PMH of seizure disorder controlled with phenobarbital (last seizure was 15 years ago), hypothyroidism controlled with Synthroid, and a recent URI. She was on a day outing with her family, slipped and fell, landing on the back of her head. She experienced a loss of consciousness at the scene. She was taken to a local hospital where a CT scan revealed a L subdural hematoma. She has been transferred to your regional medical center, which has a neurosurgeon on call.

1. The ED RN gives you the above information during a phoned report. What other information do you need to prepare for this patient?

2. Because you always have trouble remembering the layers of the brain and different hematomas, you look up subdural hematoma before S.B. arrives. What do you find?

3. S.B.'s subdural is considered acute because symptoms appeared within 24 hours of injury. What are the other classifications of subdural hematomas?

4. What are common signs and symptoms of an acute subdural hematoma?

5. Why are the elderly and alcoholics at-risk for chronic subdural hematomas?

6. How would you monitor for neurologic change?

7. Why is it especially important to make sure S.B. is taking her phenobarbital and has a therapeutic serum level?

8. The decision was made in S.B.'s case not to do a craniotomy. When would a neurosurgeon decide to treat medically vs. perform surgery?

9. Burr holes work only for acute subdurals, and a craniotomy must be done for subacute and chronic subdurals. Why?

10. Why would hypotonic IV solutions such as D_5W be avoided?

11. How would you position S.B. in bed?

12. If S.B.'s level of consciousness started to decrease, what information would you give the neurosurgeon when you call him?

13. How would you provide support to the family?

14. The neurosurgeon has ordered codeine IM as a pain medication. Why did he order codeine?

Case Study 6

R.B. is an 80-year-old English woman who is visiting a friend in the United States. One morning her friend noticed that upon awakening, R.B. had slurred speech, a R facial droop, and was disoriented. She was transported to the hospital where a CT scan confirmed the diagnosis of intracranial hemorrhage. Because of the location of the bleed, surgery was not possible and over the next couple days R.B.'s R facial droop progressed to a totally flaccid R side. R.B. was transferred to your rehabilitation facility for therapy. Ten days after the initial insult, R.B. still has some confusion, memory problems, difficulty swallowing, slurred speech, and profound R sided weakness. She is hoping to be able to return to England soon.

1. Define CVA.

2. List 3 main causes of a CVA and describe how they disrupt the O_2 supply.

3. List 10 factors that increase the risk of a CVA.

4. What is the overall goal of rehabilitation?

5. List 12 potential members of the rehabilitation health care team.

6. Why is positioning with proper body alignment so important for a patient like M.E.?

7. An aggressive exercise program must be part of the rehabilitative process to maintain and improve muscle tone and function and to prevent further disability. Describe the following exercise classifications: passive, active, active assistive, active resistive, and isometric.

8. What are some nursing interventions for R.B. related to the patient problem of weight loss r/t continued swallowing problems and risk for aspiration r/t swallowing difficulty.

9. Discharge planning begins upon admission to any facility. What special discharge needs does R.B. have and who needs to be involved?

Once the family is located and contacted, the nurse and the physician should talk to them. Offer to have a physician from the receiving facility in England call and talk to the discharging physician from your institution. FAXes are a common way of communicating from the United Kingdom to the U.S.

10. R.B. seems to be homesick. What nursing interventions could you plan to help her homesickness?

Case Study 7

You are assigned to take care of M.X. this evening's shift. In report you are told that she is a 40-year-old obese (112 kg) woman who arose from a sitting position and experienced acute and severe low back pain 3 weeks ago. She was diagnosed with herniated disks L4-S1. Dr. W., who performed a lumbar laminectomy 3 days ago, is concerned because her WBC count has gone from 8.1 mm^3 to 19.6 mm^3.

1.   What is meant by the term *herniated disk* (herniated nucleus pulposus)?

2.   What tests may be performed to detect and diagnose the herniation?

3.   What is a laminectomy?

4.   Identify 2 general objectives of postoperative nursing care of M.X.?

5.   What is meant by "log-rolling?"

6.   You ask 4 coworkers to help you log-roll M.X. As one nurse enters the room she makes a statement about breaking her back trying to move M.X. You are a little overweight yourself and watch M.X.'s face when she hears the remark. How would you handle the situation?

7.   Patients who have undergone a lumbar laminectomy frequently experience paralytic ileus and urinary retention. Why?

8. What are 4 possible sources of infection that may account for M.X.'s elevated WBC?

9. M.X. asks you how you would know if her wound were infected. Differentiate between signs and symptoms of wound infection for M.X.

10. Discharge planning should begin the day M.X. is admitted to your unit. What factors should discharge planning include?

11. List 7 written home care instructions that should be reviewed and given to M.X. before discharge.

M.X. was treated with aggressive antibiotic therapy for a urinary tract infection (UTI). With the help and support of her family, M.X. was discharged to home where she made a complete recovery. After talking to you, M.X. started on a healthy low-fat diet and lost 52 pounds over the next 9 months. When you were arranging her discharge papers, you discovered that M.X. was a script writer for soap operas! Six months after her discharge, she calls to meet you for coffee. She asks if you would like to supplement your income by consulting with her on improving the image of nurses in soap operas. She said it was your professionalism that gave her this idea.

Case Study 8

F.N. is a 57-year-old housewife, happily married with grown children, and 2 new grandchildren. F.N. made an appointment with her optometrist to explore a progressive OS visual loss over a 9-month period. Her eye exam was essentially normal, and the optometrist referred her to a neurologist. After workup, a 2.5 cm brain mass was found, and surgery was scheduled. Her only past medical history (PMH) is hypertension, for which she takes nifedipine XL 60 mg qd and potassium chloride (K-dur) 10 mEq bid, and her past surgical history (PSH) includes T&A as a child, cholecystectomy, and a TAH at age 42. She also takes a conjugated estrogen (Premarin) 0.625 mg qd.

1.   Name 4 tests that can be done to evaluate for brain tumor.

There is no standardized, universally accepted system of classifying brain tumors. They can be classified according to histologic basis, intraaxial vs. extraaxial, or malignant vs. benign.

2.   Using the term *benign* when discussing brain tumors is somewhat misleading. Why?

3.   Onset of neurologic symptoms is usually insidious, and they exhibit symptoms in relation to the area of the brain where the tumor is located. List 6 general symptoms associated with many brain tumors.

4.   Dexamethasone (Decadron) is commonly prescribed when a tumor is diagnosed and the presence of increased intracranial pressure (IICP) is demonstrated. It is administered preoperatively and postoperatively, and in conjunction with radiation and chemotherapy. Why is Decadron prescribed, and why should it not be abruptly stopped?

5. Other common supportive medications include antiseizure, diuretics, antacids and H_2 blockers, analgesics, antiemetics, and antidepressants. Indicate why each is used.

6. Once the diagnosis is made, the patient and family must be involved in the plan for treatment. Treatment depends on the type and location of the tumor and can include surgery, radiation, chemotherapy, or any combination of these. The patient also has the right to refuse treatment. Identify 4 other considerations the medical team, patient, and family will consider in devising a treatment plan.

7. Describe common responses to a diagnosis of a brain tumor.

8. List 2 role-relationship nursing diagnoses for F.N.

9. F.N. drew up a living will and health care power of attorney after she heard the diagnosis. She also sat down with her family and made her wishes known. Why is this important for F.N. in particular and for everyone in general?

10. You enter F.N.'s room to take VS and she says, "What if I come out of surgery and I'm different? Or what if I die? My grandbabies will never know me." You hear the concern in her voice. Suggest several ways that F.N. can communicate with her loved ones in the event that her surgery is unsuccessful.

11. F.N. had the surgery and was admitted to ICU postop. She did very well and remained neurologically intact (q1h neuro checks), her BP was slightly elevated (147/68), the rest of her VS were normal, she had 2 peripheral IVs, TED hose, O_2 at 4 L/nc, and a Foley. Postoperatively, F.N.'s K level dropped to 2.7 mEq/L and glucose was 202 mg/dl. Describe possible reasons why these 2 laboratory values are abnormal, and identify what treatment will be ordered to correct each.

F.N. did suffer mild neurologic damage as a result of the surgery. She was discharged to a rehabilitation facility, and eventually was able to recover most of her lost function. She continues to enjoy an active life, and has become involved in helping others facing similar experiences.

For additional information contact:
Brain Injury Association Help Line
1776 Massachusetts Ave. N.W., Suite 100
Washington, DC 20036
1-800-444-6443

Case Study 9

You walk in to T.E.'s room on initial rounds and find Mrs. E. in tears. She says, "He is having such a rough time, I wonder if I'll ever have the same man back." You heard in report that T.E. is a 63-year-old man who, while at breakfast with his wife several days ago, developed slurred speech, became severely confused, and collapsed to his R side. The acute episode began resolving in approximately 15 minutes while en route to the ED. Mrs. E. was almost hysterical because her husband had had 2 episodes of "being revived from sudden cardiac death" 5 years ago. A CT scan revealed an acute L middle cerebral aneurysm (frontal/parietal) stroke. Heparin therapy was started right away and the next day an angiogram revealed high grade L carotid artery stenosis with very stagnant flow. The heparin was discontinued, and he was taken to the OR for a carotid endarterectomy. After 2 days in the ICU, he is on your floor. T.E. has R-sided paralysis and expressive aphasia.

1. What is an angiogram and why was it important to perform an angiogram in T.E.'s case?

2. Describe a carotid endarterectomy.

3. Because T.E. already suffered a CVA, why is the carotid endarterectomy being performed?

4. Why is a baseline neurologic exam extremely important for T.E.?

5. T.E.'s current VS are 128/78, 88 (irregularly irregular), 18, 35.8°C (O), and SaO_2 of 96% on 6 L O_2/nc. Are you concerned about any of these numbers and if so why?

6. You call the ICU nurse to ask her about the irregular heart rate. She says that he was in a normal sinus rhythm while in the NICU and adds, "It wouldn't be too good if he flipped into A-fib." She suggested calling the physician. What are you going to tell the physician when you call him? What test do you expect him to prescribe?

7. Why is atrial fibrillation of concern?

8. Identify 4 nursing interventions that may improve his oxygenation and decrease T.E.'s O_2 requirements.

9. You wonder if T.E. truly requires 6 L O_2/nc because you continually find his nasal cannula pulled down onto his lip. When you ask him about moving the tubing, he states that it is irritating the inside of his nose. What can you do to decrease the irritability of the high-flow oxygen?

10. The following is a list of T.E.'s medications. Indicate why he is receiving each.
    *   Albuterol 2.5 mg nebulized q4h:

    *   Heparin sodium 5000 U SQ q12h:

    *   Multivitamin 1 cap PO AM:

    *   Nicotine 14 mg top patch qd:

    *   Nystatin suspension 4 ml PO tid:

    *   Psyllium/Sod. Bicarb. 1 packet powder PO tid:

    *   Ranitidine 150 mg PO bid:

    *   Ticlopidine 250 mg PO bid:

11. Mrs. E. is not coping well with her husband's illness. What measures could be taken to support her?

12. You find yourself speaking very loudly to T.E. due to his expressive aphasia. Your coworker admits she does the same thing when she has patients with expressive aphasia. Why don't you need to speak loudly and what are some ways to enhance communication with this patient?

T.E. was eventually discharged home with some residual expressive aphasia.

Case Study 10

You are working at a skilled nursing facility that cares for patients on ventilators. G.W. is your first patient with Guillain-Barré syndrome. G.W. is a divorced, self-supporting 56-year-old woman from a small town who developed a URI after caring for her grandson who had the same. Three weeks later she developed weakness, numbness, and tingling in her feet that progressed up her body. Her physician recognized the seriousness of her condition and transferred her to a tertiary referral center. Within days she became totally paralyzed; she was trached and placed on mechanical ventilation. She spent 1 month in the neuro critical care unit and several months on the floor before being transferred to your facility. Her only inhospital complication was pneumonia, which has totally resolved. The physicians don't know how long the paralysis will last.

1. What adaptations would you or your family have to make if you were paralyzed and unable to perform your normal responsibilities? How would you feel if you were totally dependent on others for your simplest needs? *Use a separate sheet of paper for a detailed response* and include daily care; financial issues, such as who would pay the rent/house note, groceries, utilities, mounting medical bills; social issues, such as who would care for your children, see to their education, meet their emotional needs; self-perception; emotions; etc.

2. Is G.W.'s case typical?

3. Why does potentially fatal respiratory dysfunction occur?

4. Describe a plan for pulmonary hygiene for G.W.

5. How do you anticipate that G.W.'s nutritional needs are being met?

6. Describe nursing interventions to manage bladder and bowel elimination for G.W.

7. What are some things you can do to decrease G.W.'s fear and anxiety?

8. You are using your expert nursing skills to avoid complications. List 4 potential complications.

9. What measures can be taken to prevent pressure ulcers?

An additional 3 weeks have passed. G.W. has recovered gross movement of her arms and some respiratory effort. She is still on a ventilator but she has gone from controlled to assisted breathing. This morning G.W. receives a letter from her health insurance company informing her that she has exceeded her lifetime limit and has been dropped from their plan. She is crying hysterically and is choking because of the increased mucous production in her sinuses. Remember that she cannot wipe her eyes or blow her nose to clear it.

10. What can be done for her?

It took G.W. almost 11 months to recover enough to be discharged to home with the assistance of a home health aide.

Case Study 11

Name: _____ *Class/Group:* _____ *Date:* _____

Instructions: All questions apply to this case study. Your response should be brief and to the point. Adequate space has been provided for answers. When asked to provide several answers, they should be listed in order of priority or significance. Do not assume information that is not provided. Please print or write legibly.

T.W. is a 22-year-old man who fell 50 feet from a chairlift while skiing and landed on hard-packed snow. He was found to have a T10-11 fracture with paraplegia. He was initially admitted to the SICU and placed on high-dose steroids for 24 hours. He was taken to surgery 48 hours postaccident for spinal stabilization. He spent 2 additional days in the SICU, 5 days on the floor, and now is ready to be transferred to your rehab unit. He continues to have no movement of his lower extremities.

1. The goal of treatment in the acute phase of spinal cord injury (SCI) is to help T.W. survive the injury and maintain physiologic stability through the period of spinal shock. Once the acute phase is over, T.W. moves into the postacute and early rehab phases. What are the treatment goals for T.W. in these phases?

2. Considering a hierarchy of rehabilitative needs for patients like T.W., number the following from highest (1) to lowest (5) priority.
   ___ Community integration and employment.
   ___ Accomplishment of self-care and ADLs.
   ___ Self-actualization.
   ___ Stabilization of the physiologic systems.
   ___ Adjustment to living at home.

3. T.W. received high-dose steroid therapy every 24 hours then he was placed on a smaller maintenance dose. What effect will steroids have on T.W.?

4. List 3 critical potential infections that T.W. should be monitored for throughout his hospitalization?

A person with an SCI at the T2-12 level should be independent in a wheelchair and able to manage ADL, including bowel and bladder care.

5. T.W. is on vitamin C 1 g PO qid. What is the purpose of this?

You request a consultation with a registered dietitian because you realize that T.W. needs proteins for healing; however, too much can stress his kidneys. The RD will adjust his diet to ensure adequate amount of protein, carbohydrates, calcium, magnesium, and zinc.

6. Rehabilitation teaching includes teaching T.W. how to manage his urinary drainage system. What would this teaching include?

7. What is the usual amount of time for the return of reflex function of the bladder?

8. The large bowel musculature has its own neural center that can directly respond to distention caused by fecal material. This is what allows most SCI patients to regain bowel control. What dietary instructions are important for T.W.?

9. T.W. should also be taught bowel training techniques. What would this teaching include?

10. What medications can assist with a bowel program?

11. Describe digital stimulation.

12. T.W. asks you if he'll ever be able to have sex again. What do you tell him and what are some possible referrals?

For patients with lesions at T6 or above, there is the potential for autonomic dysreflexia (AD) in response to noxious stimulation of the sympathetic nervous system. The patient develops severe hypertension (as high as 240-300/150 mm Hg), pounding headache, bradycardia, blurred vision, nausea, nasal congestion, and flushing and sweating above the level of the injury and goose bumps or pallor below the level of the injury. Potential causes include bladder distention, obstruction, infection, spasms, catheterization, and bladder irrigations done too fast or with cold fluid; bowel constipation, impaction, or rectal stimulation; and alterations in skin integrity including pressure, infection, injury, and cold or hot. This can cause retinal hemorrhage, CVA, and seizure activity.

13. What are nursing interventions r/t AD?

For additional information contact:
    National Spinal Cord Injury Association
    545 Concord Ave, Suite 29
    Cambridge, MA 02138
    1-800-962-9629

Case Study 12

Name: _____ *Class/Group:* _____ *Date:* _____

Instructions: All questions apply to this case study. Your response should be brief and to the point. Adequate space has been provided for answers. When asked to provide several answers, they should be listed in order of priority or significance. Do not assume information that is not provided. Please print or write legibly.

R.P. is 72 years old, retired, and in good health. His only medication is an aspirin a day. While bending over to tie his shoes, R.P. developed a severe headache, muscle rigidity, slurred speech, confusion, and nausea. He was taken to the ED, where it was discovered that he had a subarachnoid hemorrhage from a ruptured grade III cerebral aneurysm. The aneurysm was surgically repaired 15 days ago, and R.P. is now being transferred to your unit.

In addition, you receive the following report. R.P. is alert and maintains eye contact but is aphasic. He does withdraw from painful stimuli and plantar reflexes bilaterally. His cardiovascular system is stable, and he has a L peripheral IV that is heparin-locked and bilateral TED hose. He is on 2 L O_2/nc and has scattered coarse breath sounds with a weak cough effort. His abdomen is distended but he does have bowel sounds in all 4 quadrants; his tube feeding is at 80 ml/h. Last bowel movement (BM) is unknown. He has a Foley to down drain and his groin skin folds are a little reddened. There is no other skin breakdown. He gets out of bed (OOB) to the total lift chair bid and tolerates it well.

1.   What other information would you like to have?

2.   R.P.'s medications are listed below. Explain why he is getting each.
   •   Heparin 5000 Units SC q12h:

   •   Metoprolol (Lopressor) 50 mg per feeding tube bid:

   •   Clonidine 0.2 mg topical patch q week:

   •   Tylenol 650 mg per feeding tube q4h prn:

   •   Temazepam (Restoril) 15 mg per feeding tube q hs prn:

   •   MOM 30 ml per feeding tube prn:

3.   Current VS are 150/85, 82, 18, 37.8°C (ear), and reported as stable. Do any of the VS concern you?

4.   What laboratory tests would be indicated for the daily draw?

5.   What are nursing interventions related to R.P.'s pulmonary hygiene?

6.   What additional information given in or omitted from report is of concern to you?

7.   If R.P.'s neurologic status started to deteriorate, what test would you anticipate the physician ordering?

8.   Lab results the next morning are: Na 140 mEq/L, K 4.2 mEq/L, Cl 100 mEq/L, CO_2 26 mEq/L, BUN 20 mg/dl, creatinine 1.2 mg/dl, glucose 107 mg/dl, WBC 12 mm^3, Hgb 13.4 g/dl, Hct 37.6%, platelets 184 mm^3. Do these concern you, and what might it indicate?

9.   What are potential sites of infection for R.P.?

10. Identify 2 nursing interventions that address R.P.'s groin redness.

Case Study 13

Name: _____ Class/Group: _____ Date: _____

Instructions: All questions apply to this case study. Your response should be brief and to the point. Adequate space has been provided for answers. When asked to provide several answers, they should be listed in order of priority or significance. Do not assume information that is not provided. Please print or write legibly.

Y.W. is a 23-year-old male student from Thailand studying electrical engineering at the university. He was ejected from a moving vehicle which was traveling 70 mph. His injuries included a severe closed head injury with an occipital hematoma, bilateral wrist fractures, and a R pneumothorax. During his NICU stay, Y.W. was intubated and placed on mechanical ventilation, had a feeding tube inserted and was placed on tube feedings, had a Foley catheter to down drain, and multiple IVs inserted. He developed pneumonia 1 month after admission.

1. Describe the term *primary head injury*.

2. Describe *secondary head injury*.

3. Why is increased intracranial pressure (IICP) so clinically important, and what are 5 signs and symptoms?

4. List 4 medication classifications and 8 nursing measures that the ICU nurses could use to control or decrease the ICP?

5. Y.W.'s medication list included clindamycin 150 mg per feeding tube q6h, ranitidine (Zantac Elixir) 150 mg per feeding tube bid, and phenytoin (Dilantin) 100 mg IVPB tid. Indicate why he is on each.

6. A STAT portable CXR was ordered after each central venous catheter (CVC) was inserted. According to hospital protocol, no one is permitted to infuse anything through the catheter until the CXR has been read by the physician or radiologist. What is the purpose of the CXR, and why isn't fluid infused through the catheter until after the CXR is read?

Yin spent 2 months in acute care and is now on your rehab unit. He follows commands but tends to get very agitated with too much stimulation. His trach site is well healed and the pneumonia is finally resolving. He is still receiving supplemental tube feeding and has some continued incontinence of both bowel and bladder. Y.W. has a very supportive group of friends who are students at the University, several of them are also from Thailand.

7. Y.W.'s latest lab results are as follows, Na 149 mEq/L, K 4.2 mEq/L, Cl 119 mEq/L, CO_2 21 mEq/L, BUN 12 mg/dl, creatinine 1.2 mg/dl, glucose 123 mg/dl, WBC 15.4 mm^3, Hgb 14.9 g/dl, Hct 36.4%, platelets 140 mm^3. Are any of these of concern to you, and what would you suggest to correct them?

8. Are you surprised by Y.W.'s agitated behavior? Explain.

9. Outline a general rehabilitation plan for Y.W. based on the above data.

10. Y.W.'s mother has just arrived in the U.S. and speaks no English. What measures can be taken to facilitate communication between medical personnel and his mother?

11. Y.W.'s mother will need a place to stay while in the U.S. What can you do to facilitate the initial contact with the Thai community?

12. What special discharge planning considerations are there in this case?

For additional information contact:
    Brain Injury Association Help Line
    1776 Massachusetts Ave. N.W., Suite 100
    Washington, DC 20036
    1-800-444-6443

Case Study 14

G.B.'s family reports that he has had progressive back pain since his decompression laminectomy 4 months ago and is now unable to walk. He has become increasingly confused over the past 2 weeks, is occasionally SOB, and is now unable to care for himself. He looks dehydrated and possibly septic. G.B. is very angry at being brought to the hospital and states, "I had this back worked on 4 months ago and I don't intend to have it done again!!" G.B. is 72 years old and had multiple health problems including GI hemorrhages, hypertension (HTN), elevated glucose, chronic lymphocytic leukemia (CLL), a remote history of kidney stones, an appendectomy, shrapnel from WW II, and a fx R femur from a mining accident. His family reports that G.B. was allergic to penicillin as a child but cannot remember what reaction he experienced.

1. Based on the information given above, review the following list of admission orders. Place an "I" by each inappropriate order and state why it is inappropriate.
    ___ Routine VS.
    ___ Routine neuro checks.
    ___ Up ad lib.
    ___ CBC, Chem 7, urinalysis, ABG, PT, PTT.
    ___ O_2 to keep SaO_2 greater than 90%.
    ___ IV $D_5\frac{1}{2}$ NS with 20 mEq of KCl/L at 100 ml/h.
    ___ NPO.
    ___ Cefazolin (Kefzol) 1 g IV q8h.
    ___ Ranitidine (Zantac) 50 mg IV q8h.
    ___ Codeine 30 mg IM q4-6h prn for pain.
    ___ Droperidol (Inapsine) 0.25 ml IV q8h prn for nausea.
    ___ Acetaminophen (Tylenol) 650 mg PO q4-6h prn for fever.
        <u>Inappropriate Orders</u>

2. Admission VS are 165/85, 76, 20, 36.7°C. Do any of the VS concern you? Explain.

3. You get the following lab results, Na 132 mEq/L, K 3.7 mEq/L, Cl 98 mEq/L, CO_2 27 mEq/L, BUN 13 mg/dl, creatinine 0.6 mg/dl, glucose 138 mg/dl, WBC 36 mm^3, Hgb 10.8 g/dl, Hct 31.3%, platelets 130 mm^3. You call the physician to report them. What orders do you anticipate in regard to a change in IV solution?

4. What part of G.B.'s PMH is consistent with the CBC results?

5. What noninvasive diagnostic test might be done to determine G.B.'s problem?

6. Why would an MRI be contraindicated in G.B.'s case?

7. G.B.'s family had to leave the hospital for a short time. When you enter his room, you find him trying to climb over the siderails. What should you consider before applying a vest (Posey) or wrist restraints?

8. As the afternoon progresses, G.B.'s oxygen saturation decreases from 96% on 2 L O_2/nc to 88%. The physician orders oxygen by mask at 6 L. What are 4 nursing interventions that can help improve his oxygenation status?

9. Diagnostic tests reveal that G.B. has an epidural abscess near his laminectomy incision, and he is scheduled for surgery. G.B. has already stated he does not plan to have any more surgery. Do you feel he is competent to make the decision? How would you proceed with obtaining consent?

The family tells the surgeon to go ahead with the surgery, against G.B.'s wishes. It was decided that he is not competent to make the decision for himself at this time.

10. What are considerations for discharge planning?

Case Study 15

D.H., a 54-year-old resort owner, has multiple chronic medical problems including type II DM for 25 years, IDDM for the past 10 years, a renal transplant 5 years ago with no signs of rejection at last biopsy, HTN, and remote peptic ulcer disease (PUD). His medications include insulin, his immunosuppressives, and 2 antihypertensives. He visited his local physician with c/o L ear, mastoid, and sinus pain. He was diagnosed with sinusitis and *Candida albicans* (thrush); cephalexin (Keflex) and nystatin (Mycostatin) were prescribed. Later that evening he developed N/V, hematemesis, and weakness, and was taken to the ED. He was admitted and started on IV antibiotics, but his condition worsened throughout the night; his dyspnea increased and he developed difficulty speaking. He was flown to your tertiary referral center and was intubated en route. On arrival, D.H. had decreased LOC with periods of total unresponsiveness, weakness, and cranial nerve deficits. His diagnosis is meningitis complicated by an aspiration pneumonia and atrial fibrillation. D.H. has continued fevers and leukocytosis despite aggressive antibiotic therapy.

1. Why is D.H. at particular risk for infection?

2. Describe bacterial meningitis.

3. What is the probable route of entry of bacteria into D.H.'s brain?

4. How do you think D.H. might have developed an aspiration pneumonia?

5. What factors influenced the physicians' decision to transport D.H. from a smaller hospital to a tertiary referral center?

6.   Name 4 tests that could be used in the diagnosis of meningitis.

7.   The following is a list of D.H's medications. Indicate next to each why he is receiving it.
   - Sliding-scale regular insulin SC.

   - Sucralfate (Carafate) 1 g per NGT q6h.

   - Azathioprine 100 mg in 100 ml D_5W IVPB qd.

   - Imipenem/cilastatin (Primaxin) 500 mg IVPB q6h.

   - Methylprednisolone (Solu-Medrol) 125 mg IV q8h.

   - Digoxin 0.125 IV qd.

   - Metronidazole (Flagyl) 500 mg IV q6h.

   - Sulfamethoxazole 800 mg/trimethoprim (Septra) 160 mg IV q12h x 15 days.

8.   The lab just called you with a glucose result of 350 mg/dl. Identify 3 factors that could contribute to D.H.'s elevated glucose level.

9.   List 7 nursing interventions for management of D.H.'s current problems.

10.   List 6 nursing interventions to prevent complications.

11. D.H.'s family is staying at a nearby motel. His adult son brings his mother to the hospital. Mrs. H. says she just wants to stay with her husband around the clock. She states, "I took care of him for 35 years now, and I'm not going to abandon him now when he needs me the most." How would you respond?

D.H.'s infection destroyed his cadaver kidney. He developed multiple system organ failure and died 7 weeks later.

Case Study 16

T.S. is a 76-year-old widower being seen in your outpatient clinic for a medication refill for his Parkinson's disease. He is a retired railroad engineer who derives great pleasure from his daily walks with his dog around his neighborhood and collecting railroad memorabilia. T.S. was diagnosed with moderate (stage III) Parkinson's disease 2 years ago. He does not smoke cigarettes or drink alcohol. His PMH includes a femur fx at age 22, a cholecystectomy at age 47, and a transurethral resection of the prostate (TURP) at age 72.

1.   Because of the interference of normal muscle tone and control of smooth muscle, patients with Parkinson's disease exhibit a classic triad of symptoms. Name them.

2.   Parkinson's is a disease of the elderly with symptoms usually first noted bxt 60-70 year olds. Why are we seeing a growing number of people with Parkinson's disease?

3.   Symptoms vary and are highly individualized. List 8 symptoms associated with Parkinson's.

Medical management of the patient with Parkinson's is usually directed toward control of symptoms with drug therapy, supportive therapy, physiotherapy, and possibly psychotherapy. Pharmacotherapy can be fairly complex in these patients because there are several types of antiparkinson drugs with different mechanisms of action. The physician works with the patient to achieve the most effective regimen and often involves trial-and-error periods.

4.   Why can't we just give oral dopamine as replacement therapy, and what medication do we give instead?

5.   Levodopa is often given in combination with carbidopa. Why?

6.   What are 5 nursing interventions to decrease the number or severity of side effects of antiparkinson medications?

7.   What advice will the registered dietitian give T.S. about his diet?

8.   T.S. asks you to explain "Parkinsonian crisis." Describe it in a way he can understand, and describe what someone should do if it occurs.

9.   If you were a home health nurse, list 6 things that you would assess to determine if T.S.'s care can be managed in his home.

10. How might T.S's PMH affect his symptoms?

For additional information, contact:
Parkinson's Disease Foundation, Inc.
650 West 168th St. or 710 W. 168th St.
New York, NY 10032
1-800-457-6676 (Toll Free)
1-212-923-4700

Case Study 17

R.G. is a 50-year-old woman who was being arrested by the police when she collapsed and had a seizure. She was transported by ambulance to the ED where a CT scan revealed a grade II subarachnoid hemorrhage (SAH). Her urine and toxicology screen were positive for cocaine, opiates, barbiturates, and benzodiazepines. The ED nurse was able to contact a son from a phone number in her purse. You are caring for R.G. 2 days postadmission. The neurosurgeons have decided to postpone surgery for 5 to 10 days because this is the time when most rebleeds occur. In the meantime, they have ordered "subarachnoid precautions."

1.   What is the purpose of subarachnoid precautions, and list 9 nursing interventions you would initiate.

2.   Describe the 5 grades of cerebral aneurysms and their criteria.

3.   Why is cerebral angiography helpful in cerebral aneurysms?

4. R.G. is very uncooperative. What psychosocial issues may be contributing to her behavior?

5. Identify 6 nursing interventions that address R.G.'s fear and anxiety.

6. The physician prescribes folic acid 0.2 ml IV qd for R.G. Why?

7. R.G. is on phenytoin (Dilantin) 100 mg PO tid and her serum Dilantin level is 7.2 μg/ml. Why is she on Dilantin, and what dose adjustment do you anticipate?

8. R.G. will be discharged with a prescription for phenytoin. In view of her previous lifestyle, list 3 main concerns with respect to this prescription. Explain.

The city released R.G. when she was admitted so the "taxpayers" wouldn't have to pay for her hospitalization. She will be transferred to a rehabilitation facility for further treatment. Her medical care will be complicated by her psychosocial and drug history.

9. List 6 essential members of the rehabilitation team who will be involved in R.G.'s care.

10. What 2 measures would be essential to include in R.G.'s discharge planning?

CHAPTER 7. ENDOCRINE DISORDERS

Case Study 1

You are volunteering at a Health Fair being conducted at a local community health clinic in a large metropolitan area. You are assigned to work with an advanced practice nurse in diabetes management and are assisting in the screening process for hyperglycemia and high WHR (waist-hip ratio). During the course of the day you meet M.M., a 42-year-old African American woman, whom you suspect has some type of diabetes mellitus. A nursing history reveals the following findings: Ht 5'6", Wt 210 lb, WHR = 0.96. M.M.'s mother, age 72, and two maternal aunts have type II diabetes mellitus (DM). M.M. has smoked 1½ packs/day of cigarettes for over 25 years and admits she should get more exercise. Screening glucose level (finger stick) is 310 mg/dl. On interview, M.M.'s only complaint is increasing fatigue over the past month and mild nocturia.

1. List the major risk factors for type II DM. Place a check mark (✓) next to the risk factors that M.M. has.
   ___ Age.
   ___ Family history.
   ___ Male pattern obesity (waist-hip ratio [WHR] > 1.0 for men and 0.8 for women).
   ___ Hispanic, African American, or Native American.

2. What is the manifestation of type II DM that M.M. has (above).

3. Identify additional data that would be necessary to arrive at a definitive diagnosis.

4. During a brief physical assessment, the practitioner checks M.M.'s eyes with an ophthalmoscope. Why?

5. M.M. tells you she has a neighbor who had to start taking insulin for diabetes after she had "bad pneumonia." Her neighbor is very thin. M.M. asks if she will need insulin and if she will lose weight like her neighbor. How would you respond to her (in plain English)?

6. M.M. tells you that she knows if she would just stop eating "sweet things" she would not have diabetes. How would you correct her understanding of the disease using understandable terminology?

7. During the interview, the nurse takes M.M.'s blood pressure and asks whether she's ever been told she has heart trouble (coronary artery disease). Explain why.

8. Discuss 2 modifiable behaviors M.M. engages in that will aggravate the pathologic effects of her type II DM.

9. M.M. agreed to come to the clinic for help; her GHb was 13%. What does this tell you about M.M.'s glucose control in the past few months?

10. Identify 3 content areas of diabetes education that are important for newly-diagnosed diabetics. Identify 3 important learning objectives for each content area.

11. Discuss 2 recommendations that you would make to individuals at the Health Fair regarding primary prevention of diabetes.

12. Explain why blood glucose testing is recommended to monitor glucose rather than urine dipstick testing.

Case Study 2

You graduated 3 months ago and are working with a home care nursing agency. Included in your caseload is J.S., a 60-year-old man suffering from chronic obstructive pulmonary disease (COPD). He has been on home oxygen, 2 L O_2/nc, for several years. Approximately 2 months ago, he was started on steroid therapy. Medications include metaproterenol (Alupent) inhaler, theophylline (Theo-Dur), terbutaline, dexamethasone, digoxin, and furosemide (Lasix). Not surprisingly, he also has a 50-pack-year history of cigarette smoking. On the way to visit J.S., you remember he has been progressively exhibiting signs/symptoms of Cushing's syndrome. You suspect J.S occasionally forgets to take his medication because he always seems to have "extra" pills in the bottle at the end of the month.

1. After you meet J.S. you begin an assessment and note the following findings. Place a check mark (✓) in the blank next to the signs/symptoms that characterize Cushing's syndrome.
    ___ Barrel chest.
    ___ Full-looking face ("moon facies").
    ___ BP 180/94.
    ___ Pursed-lip breathing.
    ___ Thin arms and legs.
    ___ Bruising on both arms.
    ___ Acne.
    ___ Diminished breath sounds.
    ___ Truncal obesity with fat around clavicles and the neck.
    ___ Weakness and fatigue.
    ___ Impaired glucose tolerance.

2. Differentiate between the cause of Cushing's syndrome and Cushing's disease.

3. Identify 3 to 4 general topics to be included in a teaching plan for J.S.

4. Identify possible consequences of suddenly stopping the dexamethasone therapy.

5. The home care nurse informs the physician of the patient's signs/symptoms. The physician decides to change J.S.'s prescription to prednisone given on alternate days. Explain the rationale for this change.

6. It is easy to forget what medications have been taken when, especially when there are several different drugs and times involved. List at least 3 ways you can help J.S. remember to take his pills as prescribed.

7. J.S. states that his appetite has increased but he is unable to satiate his appetite because of shortness of breath and he has been losing weight. How would you address this problem? How might his diet be modified?

8. You advise J.S. to take his prednisone with food and then ask him a series of questions related to his vision. Discuss the rationale behind these nursing care actions.

9. Differentiate between the glucocorticoid and mineralocorticoid effects of prednisone.

10. How would your assessment change if J.S. were taking a glucocorticoid that also has significant mineralocorticoid activity?

11. Review J.S.'s list of medications. Based on what you know about the side effects of loop diuretics and steroids, discuss the potential problem of administering these in combination with digoxin.

12. Realizing that patients like J.S. are susceptible to all types of infections, you write guidelines to prevent infections. Identify 4 major points that these guidelines will include.

Case Study 3

E.H. is a 60-year-old woman who has rheumatoid arthritis. For the past 12 years she has been taking prednisone 60 mg daily (40 mg in the AM, 20 mg in the PM), and nonsteroidal antiinflammatory drugs (NSAIDS) to control her disease and symptoms. As a result of her autoimmune disorder and/or long-term steroid use, E.H. has adrenal insufficiency. The physician adjusts her steroid dosage for replacement therapy. In your nursing role, you are asked to conduct educational sessions designed to teach E.H. about her condition and the treatment she needs.

1. E.H. states she doesn't understand how her taking steroids has caused her body to lose it's ability to produce the "the real thing." How would you explain this paradox in terms she can understand?

2. People receiving steroid replacement should be taught signs/symptoms that signal the dosage is too low. What are the signs/symptoms of inadequate steroid replacement?

3. What would you teach someone like E.H. about the nutritional implications of adrenal insufficiency?

4. Explain why the AM dosage of prednisone is higher.

5. E.H. confides in you that she is afraid of taking steroids any longer because she has read about the deleterious effects of steroid abuse by athletes. How would you counter this misconception and alleviate E.H.'s concern?

6. How would teaching differ for this patient (on replacement therapy) as compared with teaching required for the patient taking therapeutic doses of glucocorticoids?

7. The patient states she is under a lot of stress because of her son's recent diagnosis of cancer and her husband's upcoming retirement. What are the teaching implications of this information?

8. You realize that taking exogenous cortisol can result in a variety of pathophysiologic alterations often described as Cushing's syndrome. Since E.H. will be taking lifelong steroids, would you expect to see the signs/symptoms associated with Cushing's syndrome in this individual? Explain your answer.

9. What signs/symptoms should you teach E.H. to monitor that would indicate excessive drug therapy?

10. You instruct E.H. on administration of a parenteral form of hydrocortisone. Under what circumstances should she take the parenteral form of the drug?

11. What measures should E.H. take to prevent an acute episode of adrenal insufficiency?

12. E.H. tells you she never used to take pills at all. She says she hates to be "addicted to a drug." What will you tell her?

Case Study 4

You are working in a community outpatient clinic where you perform the intake assessment on R.M., a 38-year-old woman who is attending graduate school. Her chief complaint is overwhelming fatigue that is not relieved by rest. She is so exhausted she has difficulty walking to classes and studying. She has coarse, sparse scalp hair; scaly skin; slightly slurred speech; thick tongue; a hoarse voice; puffiness around the eyes; yellowish-colored skin and nails; and swollen neck. Initial VS were 92/64, 56, 12, 96.8°F (rectal).

1. Compare her VS with those of a healthy person her same age.

2. List 8 general questions you might ask R.M. to get a "ball park" idea of what is going on with her.

3. You know that *some* of R.M.'s symptoms could be caused by depression, hypothyroidism, anemia, cardiac disease, fluid and electrolyte imbalance, or allergies. As part of your screening procedures, how would you begin to investigate which of these conditions probably *do not* account for R.M.'s symptoms?

You found no obvious irregularities in R.M.'s cardiopulmonary assessment.

4. Unnecessary diagnostic tests are expensive. What tests would you think would be the most important to be obtained on R.M. and why?

After reviewing the laboratory results, the family nurse practitioner diagnoses R.M. with hypothyroidism and places her on thyroid replacement therapy.

5. The practitioner prescribes levothyroxine (Synthroid) 1.7 μg/kg body weight/day. R.M. weighs 130 lb. What should be her daily dose of Synthroid in milligrams? How would her prescription read?

    Note: Micrograms are alternately written μg or mcg.

6. R.M.'s T_3 and T_4 levels were decreased and the TSH level was increased. Explain the relationship between these lab results and hypothyroidism.

7. What patient teaching needs will you review with R.M. before she leaves? Remember medication issues.

8. Why would you want to obtain a complete drug history on R.M.?

9. What general teaching issues would you address with R.M.?

10. R.M. wonders if she should take iodine supplements if she decreases her salt intake. She recognizes that salt is a significant source of iodine in her part of the country. What would you explain to her?

11. What should you teach her regarding prevention of myxedema coma?
    *   Caution R.M. to

12. Before R.M. leaves the clinic, she asks how she will know if the medication is "doing its job." Outline simple expected outcomes for R.M.

13. Several weeks later, R.M. calls the clinic stating she can't remember if she took her thyroid medication. What additional data should you obtain, and how would you advise her?

14. Under what circumstances should R.M. hold the drug or call the clinic?

R.M. comes in 2 months later for a follow-up visit. You can't believe she is the same person. She looks and walks 10 years younger. Her skin appears more moist and her hair is beginning to come in with its normal feel. "You can't believe how much different I'm feeling," she says. "I'm discovering what it's like to live again."

Case Study 5

You are working on an oncology unit and will be receiving a client from the recovery room. The PACU (post-anesthesia care unit) nurse calls and gives the following report. C.P., a 50-year-old woman, had a total thyroidectomy (multinodular goiter), left superior and right inferior parathyroidectomy due to adenoma; the EBL (estimated blood loss) was 25 ml. VS are 130/82, 80-90, 20. She has a peripheral IV of $D_5 \frac{1}{2}$ NS with 20 mEq KCl and 10 mEq calcium gluconate infusing at 100 ml/h. She has received a total of 50 mg meperidine (Demerol) IVP and she remains alert and oriented. C.P.'s PMH includes TAH (total abdominal hysterectomy) for fibroids, and low-level radiation treatments to the neck 38 years ago for eczema. Her medications include estradiol (Estrace), lovastatin (Mecavor), and levothyroxine (Synthroid). Both parents are living; her father had an MI at 70 years old, her mother has hypothyroidism but never had thyroid tumors. Preoperative laboratory findings: calcium 11.2 mg/dl, phosphorus 2.4 mg/dl, Cl 106 mEq/L, alkaline phosphatase 112 U/L, elevated parahormone and TSH levels, creatinine 1.4 mg/dl.

1. What additional data should you obtain from the recovery room nurse?

2. What preparations will you take before C.P. arrives?

3. You receive C.P. from the recovery room. How will you focus your initial assessment and why?

4. During your initial assessment you document negative Chvostek's and Trousseau's signs. Describe data that would support this conclusion.

5. Explain why C.P. would have been taking Synthroid preoperatively.

6. Identify the major risk factor that may have contributed to the development of parathyroid adenoma in C.P.

7. Identify 4 nursing diagnoses for C.P.

8. Identify 4 nursing measures that you should include in the postoperative care of C.P.

9. Identify nursing care measures that reduce the risk for postoperative swelling.

10. The next day, 24 hours after surgery, C.P. calls you into her room complaining of numbness around her mouth and tingling at the tips of her fingers. She appears restless but is alert and oriented. Realizing that C.P. may be experiencing hypocalcemia, you decide to notify the physician. What should you do in the interim before the physician returns your call?

11. What emergency equipment should you gather?

C.P. is given supplemental calcium gluconate and recovers without further complications. C.P. is being discharged 48 hours postoperatively. She states that she can't wait until she can stop taking the Synthroid.

12. How would you respond to her statement?

Case Study 6

Name: _____ Class/Group: _____ Date: _____

Instructions: All questions apply to this case study. Your response should be brief and to the point. Adequate space has been provided for answers. When asked to provide several answers, they should be listed in order of priority or significance. Do not assume information that is not provided. Please print or write legibly.

K.B. is an 80-year-old woman admitted to the hospital following a 5-day episode of the "flu" with c/o DOE (dyspnea on exertion), palpitations, chest pain, insomnia, and fatigue. Her PMH includes CHF (congestive heart failure) and HTN (hypertension) requiring antihypertensive medications (she states that she has not been taking these medications on a regular basis). K.B. was diagnosed with Graves' disease 6 months ago and was placed on propylthiouracil (PTU) 100 mg PO q6h. Assessment findings are as follows: Ht 62", Wt 100 lb. Appears anxious and restless. Loud heart sounds; VS are 150/90, 104 irregular, 20, 100.2°F; 1+ pitting edema noted in lower extremities. Diminished breath sounds with fine crackles in the posterior bases. K.B. states she recently lost her husband. Laboratory findings: Hgb 11.8 g/dl, Hct 36%, ESR (erythrocyte sedimentation rate) 48 mm/h, Na 141 mEq/L, K 4.7 mEq/L, Cl 101 mEq/L, BUN 33 mg/dl, creatinine 1.9 mg/dl, T_4 RIA 14.0 µg/dl, T_3 230 ng/dl.

1. Of the physical assessment and laboratory findings, which represent manifestations of hypermetabolism?

2. What additional subjective and objective data would you gather for someone with Graves' disease?

3. Following AM rounds, the physician leaves the following orders. Which of the orders would you question and why?
   Propranolol (Inderal) 20 mg PO q6h.
   Dexamethasone (Decadron) 10 mg IV q6h.
   Verapamil (Calan SR) 120 mg PO qd.
   Diet as tolerated, high-protein.
   STAT ECG.
   Up ad lib.

4. Develop 4 priority nursing diagnoses for K.B.

5. Later on your shift, you note that K.B. is extremely restless and is disoriented to person, place, and time. VS are 104/62, 180 and irregular, 32 and labored, 103°F. Her ECG shows atrial fibrillation. What do these findings indicate?

6. What would you do *first*?

K.B. is in thyroid crisis. The physician orders the following: STAT ABG; digoxin (Lanoxin) 0.125 mg IVP q8h x 3 doses; IV of D_5W at 100 ml/h; Lugol's solution (strong iodine) 10 drops PO tid; increase propylthiouracil (PTU) to 200 mg PO qid; hydrocortisone (Hydro-Cort) 100 mg IVP q8h; cardiac monitor; absolute bed rest; cooling blanket for temp > 102°F; acetaminophen (Tylenol) 650 mg PO prn temp > 100°F.

7. Why did the physician order acetaminophen instead of salicylates?

8. Identify 4 nursing measures that would be essential in caring for K.B.

9. Identify 2 possible contributing factors that may have precipitated K.B.'s thyroid storm.

10. Before discharge, the physician discusses 2 treatment options with K.B. and her family: radioactive iodine therapy (RAI) using ^{131}I, and subtotal thyroidectomy. K.B. is fearful of radiation treatment and asks you for your opinion. How would you respond?

11. K.B. decides to receive ^{131}I. During pretreatment instructions, the family asks if she will be radioactive and what precautions they should take. Outline important guidelines for instructing K.B. and her family on home precautions.

12. Discuss how your discharge teaching instructions will differ from those you would give to someone following a subtotal thyroidectomy.

Case Study 7

A.R. is a 50-year-old Native American college professor (medical anthropology) with a history of Type II diabetes mellitus (NIDDM) for the past 10 years. He has been controlling his glucose by taking glyburide (Diabeta, Micronase) and using a 2000 calorie ADA (American Diabetes Association) diet. He is aware of the higher incidence of type II DM in his people and is open to anything he can learn about it. His blood glucose level had been fairly consistent with an average AM reading of 200 mg/dl. He is 74" and weighs 220 lb, having lost 10 lb over the past month. Six months after hospitalization for viral pneumonia, A.R. is readmitted for hyperglycemia. He has been running higher blood glucose levels (280 to 300 mg/dl) and has lost 10 lb. He is currently on a medical leave of absence from work. His medical history includes a myocardial infarction, hypertension, and renal insufficiency.

1. Dr. J., A.R.'s physician, determines that A.R. requires insulin for glucose control and orders regular human insulin per sliding scale before breakfast and supper; NPH human insulin 20 Units before breakfast and supper. When would you expect the regular insulin to have its peak effect compared with NPH?

2. You are aware of the new American Diabetic Association (ADA) (1994) nutrition recommendations and principles for people with diabetes mellitus (ADA, 1994). A.R.'s physician does not appear aware of these guidelines. You would like to try these guidelines on A.R. to see if he can obtain better glucose control. You know A.R.'s physician has been open to new ideas in the past as long as they have a sound, scientific basis. What collegial strategy might you use to approach him about a change in A.R.'s treatment plan?

3. What other health care professionals may be helpful to you in working out a strategy for A.R.'s care?

4. None of the other nurses on your unit knows about the more recent developments in diabetes management. Many of the patients on your floor are diabetics. What are 3 activities you can undertake to promote professional growth and development on your unit? (Be creative!)

5. A.R. says he isn't too keen on "jabbing himself with a needle a couple times a day." He wants to know why he can't keep on taking the oral insulin he has been using (glyburide). What is the basis for your response?

A.R.'s revised care plan calls for tighter glucose control with glucose levels of 80 to 120 mg/dl being the recommended range. Dr. J. has discussed with him the importance and benefit of keeping his glucose below 140 mg/dl, and you are going to talk to him about administering his insulin.

6. While you are teaching A.R. how to administer the insulin, he asks why it is necessary to prepare the regular insulin first. Offer a meaningful reason for this procedural step.

7. At 0300 A.R. calls you into his room c/o of sweating, nausea, and "shakiness." What would you do first?

It is determined that A.R.'s blood glucose is 65 mg/dl.

8. Of the following choices, indicate which item(s) would be appropriate to give A.R. to immediately treat hypoglycemia.
   ___ ½ cup pure orange juice.
   ___ 1 slice of bread.
   ___ 2 graham cracker squares.
   ___ 1 glass of milk.
   ___ Half a bagel.
   ___ ½ cup soda pop (not diet or sugar-free).

9. Of the following statements, which one(s) indicate that A.R. requires further teaching regarding self-care?

___ My wife and I enjoy soaking in our hot tub.

___ My feet get cold, and the heating pad I use sure helps.

___ I'll have to have my wife help me look at my feet since I can't see as well as I used to.

___ Sometimes I can't even feel my feet, especially if I've been sitting for a long time.

___ These thick toenails should probably be cut by a doctor.

___ This file I have works great for these calluses on my feet.

10. A.R. says he has read that exercise can help people with diabetes. Outline the benefits and risks of exercise for the diabetic patient in general. State how the risks can be minimized.

11. Develop a teaching plan that addresses the special needs of A.R. as he embarks on an exercise program. Include at least 8 points.

12. The dietitian evaluates A.R.'s eating pattern and determines his frequent hyperglycemic episodes are related to eating candy or sweet rolls during these periods and lack of knowledge regarding the difference between simple and complex carbohydrates. Offer an analogy that would help A.R. comprehend this concept.

Case Study 8

W.V., a 40-year-old woman, has been referred to the endocrine clinic of a large metropolitan medical center by her primary care physician. She presents with a history of bilateral hemianopsia, headaches, menstrual disturbances (amenorrhea), dyspareunia, and lethargy. An extensive history reveals polyuria and polydipsia. Her family physician suspects an anterior pituitary tumor. GH, prolactin, TSH, LH, and FSH levels are unremarkable. A dexamethasone suppression test (or cortisol/ACTH challenge test) and 24-hour urine for 17-hydroxysteroids (17-OHCS) are planned.

1. W.V. is aware of the high probability of a pituitary tumor but she doesn't understand why the physician wants to test her kidneys. How would you explain the relationship between the pituitary and adrenal glands and the need for adrenal function studies to her?

2. Identify 4 nursing diagnoses for W.V.

The dexamethasone suppression test was normal but the 24-hour urine for 17-OHCS was elevated. An MRI (magnetic resonance imaging) was ordered.

3. The MRI confirms a macroadenoma of the anterior pituitary. The physician advises a transsphenoidal hypophysectomy. What questions would you anticipate W.V. might have?

4. While W.V.'s physician arranges for her admission to the hospital and schedules her transsphenoidal hypophysectomy, you enter her examining room to conduct preop teaching. You find W.V. crying. She says she is embarrassed by the hormonal changes and states, "I'm afraid my husband won't love me anymore." What approaches would be appropriate for addressing the patient's fear?

5. During preop teaching, W.V. states she is fearful of the procedure. She says she doesn't understand how a tumor in the brain can be removed through the nose. How would you explain the procedure to minimize her fear?

6. Identify 2 major teaching needs for postop care based on the transsphenoidal approach. Outline important educational points for each area to address during preop teaching with W.V.

7. W.V. is admitted and undergoes a successful transsphenoidal hypophysectomy. Ten hours postop, W.V. calls her nurse into her room complaining of postnasal drip. She is frequently swallowing. What 5 actions should the nurse take and give your rationale.

8. The nurse notes the following assessment findings: VS 100/66, 98, 16; W.V. c/o thirst; her skin is flushed; her urine output 300 ml/h with a specific gravity of 1.003, and she is flaccid (e.g., no muscle tone). What additional information should you gather before calling the physician?

9. The nurse suspects fluid volume deficit related to inadequate release of ADH. While waiting for the surgeon to return her call, what should the nurse's priority intervention(s) be?

10. The surgeon orders a serum and urine osmolality and electrolytes. The lab reports a urine osmolality of 95 mOsm/kg, serum osmolality of 315 mOsm/kg, and sodium level of 146 mEq/L. Discuss the significance of each.

11. Replacement therapy for diabetes insipidus includes administration of aqueous vasopressin (Pitressin) or the synthetic vasopressin analog desmopressin (DDAVP). Compare the advantage(s) and disadvantage(s) of using desmopressin versus aqueous Pitressin in this situation.

12. How will the nurse evaluate the effectiveness of drug and fluid therapy?

Case Study 9

You are a nurse on a medical unit. One of your patients, T.L., a 40-year-old man who works as a communications supervisor, is being evaluated for uncontrolled HTN. He c/o frequent episodes of chest pain and palpitations, diaphoresis, job stress, nervousness, epigastric distress after eating, and pounding migraine headaches that leave him exhausted. He states that these episodes have increased in frequency and duration; he now experiences several episodes a week, and each episode lasts 1 to 3 days. He has taken a variety of antihypertensive medications, none of which have successfully controlled his HTN. His blood pressure is labile; sometimes it is normal and other times it is 220/120. Cardiac workup reveals no significant cardiovascular abnormalities. He has a 27-pack year smoking history. T.L.'s 24-hour urine analysis reveals: vanillylmandelic acid (VMA) 12 mg/24h; epinephrine 45 ng/24h, and norepinephrine 100 ng/24h; CT scan reveals a single adrenomedullary tumor. T.L. is diagnosed with pheochromocytoma and scheduled for an adrenalectomy.

1. The physician informs T.L. that an adrenal tumor is causing his symptoms. T.L. is obviously upset with his diagnosis. He states he doesn't understand how a tumor on top of his kidney can cause high blood pressure. He asks if this means he has cancer. How would you respond?

2. The physician advises T.L. to undergo an adrenalectomy. He is immediately started on phenoxybenzamine (Dibenzyline) 20 mg PO q8h, and propranolol (Inderal) 40 mg PO bid. What is the connection between these two drugs and the diagnosis?

3. Some people experience paroxysmal, or sudden, periodic attacks of HTN that correspond to the release of epinephrine and/or norepinephrine. Under what circumstances would T.L. most likely experience a paroxysmal hypertensive event?

4. What measures to prevent a paroxysmal hypertensive event should you teach T.L.?

5. T.L. is given hydrocortisone (Solu-Cortef) 100 mg IV push preoperatively. Discuss the significance of this drug in the preoperative period.

6. Following the surgery, T.L. is taken directly to the intensive care unit. The anesthesiologist gives the admitting nurse the following report: the surgery went well, and T.L. should wake up shortly; his VS have been running 180/90, 88, 16, 96.1 °F; he's got a left subclavian Swan-Ganz catheter and 2 large-bore peripheral IVs with D_5W running at a total of 125 ml/h; urine output during OR was 200 ml. What additional data should the ICU nurse elicit from the anesthesiologist?

7. Identify 3 postoperative nursing diagnoses for T.L.

8. For each nursing diagnoses identified above, outline 2 to 3 nursing measures.

9. During shift assessment (second postop day), the nurse notes that T.L. seems less alert, his grip strength is markedly weaker than yesterday, and his mucous membranes are dry. The previous nurse reported that he had vomited twice in the last hour. The cardiac monitor shows peaked T waves and a widened QRS complex. VS are 120/72, 94, 14, 101 °F. What conclusions can you draw from the above data?

All of these findings suggest adrenal insufficiency.

10. Based on the nurses' assessment findings, what general treatment measures would you anticipate?

11. Outline 4 nursing care measures that are critical during this period.

12. T.L. is stabilized and is scheduled to be discharged to home. During discharge teaching, T.L. asks if he will require steroids for the rest of his life. How should you respond to T.L.?

Case Study 10

You are a hospice nurse caring for G.N., a 40-year-old man diagnosed with oat cell carcinoma of the lung with widespread metastasis. He is receiving morphine sulfate (MS Contin) 30 mg PO q6h for chronic pain management, prednisone (Deltasone) 10 mg PO qd, and is on 2 L O_2/nc. He is currently undergoing radiation treatments for palliative relief of shoulder and chest pain. At the weekly patient care conference, you and the physician discuss the possibility that G.N. is experiencing SIADH (syndrome of inappropriate antidiuretic hormone) related to his tumor. G.N. and his wife desire only comfort measures; they are against hospitalization and all means of artificial life support.

1. How would you differentiate between the onset of SIADH and the side effects of radiation, morphine, or prednisone therapy?

During your daily assessment, you note that G.N. is complaining of increased nausea and malaise. He has gained 5 pounds over the last 3 days without signs of edema, and his urine appears to be more concentrated. His wife states he has been sleeping a lot more lately. After consulting with the physician, you draw blood for a serum sodium level and deliver the blood to the laboratory for analysis.

2. The laboratory reports a serum Na of 122 mEq/L. Explain why individuals with SIADH-induced total body water gain generally do not have the hypernatremia and dependent edema that is commonly seen in congestive heart failure and cirrhosis of the liver.

3. During collaboration, you and the physician discuss the treatment plan of restricting fluids to 500 ml/d and increasing the oral salt intake to raise G.N.'s serum sodium level. As you analyze G.N.'s total clinical picture, is there reason to question this plan of action?

4. G.N.'s wife asks how she can help her husband adhere to the fluid restriction when he seems to be so thirsty. What strategies can you offer her?

5. Two days later, G.N.'s wife calls to inform you that her husband is vomiting, is disoriented to time and place, and c/o severe headache. What will you do first?

6. The physician explains the situation to G.N.'s wife, and she agrees to have her husband transported to the ED for IV administration of sodium chloride and diuretics. You call the ED to inform the staff of G.N.'s arrival. What information should you convey to the triage nurse?

7. The ED physician prescribed the following: start an IV of 3% sodium chloride and infuse 100 ml over 1 hour; then draw STAT serum Na, Cl, HCO_3, and osmolality and send urine for osmolality. Administer furosemide (Lasix) 40 mg IV push. Discuss the possible consequences of too rapid infusion of the saline solution.

8. When should the Lasix be given? Explain.

9.   Identify priority assessment parameters the ED nurse should monitor during this
     acute period.

10. Upon discharge from the ED, the physician orders demeclocycline (Declomycin).
     Analyze the high-risk side effects of democlocylcine for G.N.

11. Outline important teaching guidelines r/t demeclocycline therapy that you would
     address with G.N. and his wife.

Case Study 11

Name: _____ Class/Group: _____ Date: _____

Instructions: All questions apply to this case study. Your response should be brief and to the point. Adequate space has been provided for answers. When asked to provide several answers, they should be listed in order of priority or significance. Do not assume information that is not provided. Please print or write legibly.

P.W. is a 40-year-old disabled man who recently lost his wife to metastatic breast cancer. His brother has taken him into his home. P.W. has a 22-year history of insulin-dependent diabetes mellitus (IDDM, now called type I diabetes mellitus). Until recently, he has taken responsibility for the management of his disease and has been actively involved in the local chapter of the American Diabetic Association. PMH includes 2 amputated toes on his R foot, retinopathy and visual impairment in both eyes, and angina on exertion from coronary artery disease that severely restricts his activity. Since he began treatment with an ace-inhibitor 2 years ago, his blood pressure has gone from 182/128 to 126/78 mm Hg. Currently, he is 71" tall and weighs 135 lb. P.W.'s sister-in-law, who is an LVN/LPN, says P.W. has lost about 12 pounds in the past 3 weeks. Over the past few years, P.W. has been administering a multidose (3 injections) regimen of regular human insulin to himself (1 before each meal and 1 injection of NPH human insulin at bedtime. Recently his blood glucose levels have been increasingly inconsistent and labile, and he has been labeled "noncompliant." It is Monday. You are the home care nurse assigned to visit P.W. 3 times per week for teaching and evaluation. P.W.'s brother and sister-in-law express concern that P.W. seems to be indifferent about his nutritional and pharmacologic regimens.

1. List measures you normally would address in teaching for both hypoglycemia and hyperglycemia (6 each).
    *   *Hyperglycemia:*

    *   *Hypoglycemia:*

Note: Current practice promotes tighter glucose management to prevent long-term complications of DM. In the past, patients' glucose often would be allowed to swing to 180 mg/dl or higher. These are the current recommendations for glucose:

1. Blood glucose levels of 60-120 mg/dl preprandial and 180 mg/dl 1 hour postprandial (Hollander, Castle, Joynes, & Nelson, p. 11, 1990).

2. The general goal is 70-120 mg/dl (as close to "normal" as possible). At this level, HbA_{1c} should be about 6% over time. Normal values for adults/elderly should be about 4% to 8%. For rough estimates of glucose levels over a period of weeks, consider an HbA_{1c} of 6% to be equal to 110 mg/dl and an HbA_{1c} of 10% to be about 250 mg/dl (Hollander et al., p. 11, 1990).

3. It may take weeks, months, or even more than a year to reach these goals safely, but it can be done (Hollander et al., p. 12, 1990). To try to reduce blood glucose levels too quickly, risks repeated hypoglycemic reactions and the frustration (as well as danger) of the Somogyi phenomenon.

4. HbA_{1c} should be done at the beginning of a risk modification program and repeated on a 4 to 8 week basis until the value is stable. Note that this value will change more slowly and be more stable, over time, than blood glucose levels.

Also note that the new 1995 American Diabetic Association guidelines are more flexible than the former guidelines and accommodate carbohydrate counting or exchanges. Current exchange lists have been published by the American Diabetes Association and the American Dietetic Association, under the title *Exchange Lists for Meal Planning*. This and other information may be obtained from the American Dietetic Association, Chicago, IL, Products and Services Division, 1-800-877-1600x5000, FAX 1-312-899-4899.

In the past, some urinary glucose and ketones often were tested at home by dipstick. Although some adults still use this method of "controlling" their disease because of habit or limited financial resources, it is grossly inaccurate. Blood glucose monitoring is the recommended method for controlling type I DM. For gestational diabetes management, consult recent authoritative sources.

As you start to review the above measures with P.W., you notice he already seems aware of what he should do to control his blood glucose. You also are concerned that he seems to be distracted and "drifts off" in the middle of a discussion; his affect also appears flat.

2. You take P.W.'s resting vital signs and get the following: 174/108, 82, 20, 98.4°F (oral). Are these values acceptable? If not, indicate which one(s) are not and what you think is happening.

You ask P.W. if he has been taking all his medications. He says "Yes" but adds that he discovers "extra" blood pressure pills left over at the end of each week. He seems to be confused about the reason for the "leftover" pills. You decide to do a glucose stick. He registers 348 mg/dl.

3.   Based on all the above information, what 2 other assessments will you want to perform on P.W.?

4.   You decide to call P.W.'s physician. Specifically, what information are you going to give her?

P.W.'s physician says she wants to hospitalize him for evaluation and stabilization; this also would give the opportunity for a psychiatric consult. P.W. says he refuses to go to "that hospital where my wife died." In discussion with P.W. and the physician, it is decided that you will check on his progress daily; someone from the home care agency will call q8h for a progress report. P.W.'s sister-in-law agrees to monitor his blood glucose and vital signs and see that he takes all his medications. If P.W.'s condition does not improve or becomes worse, he must enter the hospital for treatment. The physician agrees with you about his being depressed and starts P.W. on sertraline (Zoloft) 50 mg qd to be taken with his bedtime snack for his depression.

5.   The next day, during your midafternoon visit to P.W.'s home, he tells you he has a headache and is feeling "fidgety." His pulse is 124, his gait is unsteady, speech is slightly slurred, and blood glucose is 48 mg/dl. What will you do?

6.   In an effort to determine the cause of this hypoglycemic reaction, what questions should you ask his sister-in-law?

7.   You ask the sister-in-law who gave him his insulin injections today: did he administer it himself, or did she? You also ask her to check the insulin vial to see if some insulin appears to be unaccounted for. Explain your rationale.

8. If P.W. were to become unconscious during a hypoglycemic episode, how would you revise nursing management of his condition in this setting?

9. P.W.'s sister-in-law phones you on Sunday morning stating that P.W. is "very sick." What questions would you ask her to help you decide the best course of action?

10. Under what circumstances is P.W. likely to experience diabetic ketoacidosis?

P.W.'s sister-in-law informs you that his blood glucose is too high for the machine to read. You tell her to dial 911 immediately; advise her to tell them P.W. is diabetic and his blood glucose is over 400 mg/dl.

11. What can the ED nurse do to prepare for P.W.'s arrival?

12. The nurse does a quick assessment upon arrival. Outline essential components of an abbreviated assessment specific for this situation.

13. Laboratory tests reveal the following: Na 135 mEq/L, K 5.6 mEq/L, Cl 92 mEq/L, BUN 38 mg/dl, glucose 682 mg/dl, WBC 15.7 mm^3, Hct 53%, pH 7.30, PaCO$_2$ 36 mm Hg, PaO$_2$ 86 mm Hg, and HCO$_3$ 18 mEq/L. Interpret the lab values in relation to this situation.

14. Write 3 nursing diagnoses that depict the care priorities for this situation.

15. The physician prescribes an IV drip per infusion pump of regular human insulin 100 units in 100 ml NS at 6 U/h for blood glucose >300 mg/dl, hourly glucose check, repeat electrolytes and serum glucose in 2 hours. What effect should the insulin infusion have on the client's physical condition and how should the nurse revise the physical assessment plan?

16. Following the DKA episode, for which P.W. was hospitalized, P.W. shares with his nurse, "I don't have the will to go on living without my wife...I wish everyone would just let me die." How should the nurse respond?

A few days later, when you visit P.W. to facilitate his discharge, you find the combination of antidepressant and improved health status has contributed to an improvement in P.W.'s mental status. He impresses you as being alert and intelligent. Although he verbalizes a sense of great loss and sadness about his wife's death, he no longer seems to be so overwhelmed. He says he has not heard about the 1994 American Diabetes Association nutrition recommendations and principles for people with diabetes mellitus and expresses interest in learning "as much as he can." You chart that he appears to be open and receptive to teaching about management of his condition. You make a mental note to yourself that a "noncompliant" patient often is a person in trouble who needs help, not a label.

CHAPTER 8. IMMUNOLOGIC DISORDERS

Case Study 1

Name: _____ Class/Group: _____ Date: _____

Instructions: All questions apply to this case study. Your response should be brief and to the point. Adequate space has been provided for answers. When asked to provide several answers, they should be listed in order of priority or significance. Do not assume information that is not provided. Please print or write legibly.

You are a nurse at the student health center (SHC) at a local university. T.Q., a 19-year-old male student, visits the clinic the first day of Autumn Quarter to inform you of his immunodeficiency problem. He gives you a letter from his attending physician, a vial of gamma globulin, and asks you if you would give him his "shot." The letter, written by T.Q.'s physician, states that he was diagnosed with primary immunodeficiency disease 4 years ago. He has an adequate number of B-cells but inadequate numbers of immunoglobulin. T.Q. has a history of chronic sinus and upper respiratory tract infections and occasional GI tract infections. He is maintained on 0.66 ml/kg gamma globulin IM every 3 weeks. T.Q. responds well to his treatment and has suffered no side effects from gamma globulin other than occasional redness at the injection site. T.Q. has no other known illnesses or allergies and is on tetracycline for acne. T.Q. is 5'11', weights 190 lb, has several pustular lesions on his face and neck, and his VS are 134/78, 84, 20, 98.8°F.

1. What actions will you take first?

2. What should you do while the physician is verifying information?

3. Would you give T.Q. his own medication?

4. What other assessments should you make before T.Q. leaves?

5. You note on T.Q.'s health record that he has not received his polio, measles, mumps, or rubella vaccines. What explanation can be given for the lack of these vaccinations?

T.Q. is very knowledgeable about his condition. After receiving his injection, he makes an appointment to return to student health in 3 weeks. T.Q. complains of a stuffy nose on his next appointment.

6. How should you respond to T.Q.'s complaints?

7. If T.Q. is developing a sinus infection, what signs are you likely to encounter upon examining T.Q.?

T.Q.'s nares do not appear swollen or red, although he does have some clear mucus drainage. His temperature is normal at 98.4°F. T.Q. is due for his next injection of gamma globulin.

8. Should you give the medication or ask him to return when he is no longer having nasal stuffiness? Why or why not?

9. Should any adjustments be made in T.Q.'s class schedule or activities because of his condition?

10. How do primary immunodeficiencies differ from secondary immunodeficiencies?

11. Explain why T.Q. is at greater risk for the development of infections than his classmates.

12. How do injections of gamma globulin help T.Q. fight off infections?

13. What are the major side effects that could occur from injections of gamma globulin?

14. Given the nature of and side effects associated with gamma globulin, how long should T.Q. wait at the health center before leaving?

Case Study 2

You are working at a physician's office where you have just taken C.Q., a 38-year-old woman, into the consultation room. C.Q. has been divorced for 5 years, has 2 daughters (ages 14 and 16), and works full-time as a legal secretary. Two weeks ago she visited her doctor for a routine physical examination and requested that an HIV (human immunodeficiency virus) test be performed. C.Q. stated that she was in a serious relationship, is contemplating marriage, and just wanted to make certain she was "Okay." No abnormalities were noted during C.Q.'s physical examination and blood was drawn for routine blood chemistries, hematology studies, and an ELISA (enzyme-linked immunosorbent assay) test, also knows as the EIA (enzyme immunoassay) test. C.Q. is at the office to receive her lab results. The physician informs you that C.Q.'s EIA was positive.

1.   What is an EIA test? Does a positive EIA mean that C.Q. definitely has HIV?

2.   You explain to C.Q. that one of her tests needs to be repeated and you need to draw another blood sample. Why wouldn't you tell C.Q. that her first test result was positive and that another test is needed before the diagnosis can be confirmed?

The physician informs you that C.Q.'s Western blot test results confirm that she is HIV positive and requests that you be present when he talks to her. Before leaving C.Q.'s room, the physician requests that you obtain another blood sample for further testing, give C.Q. verbal and written information about local AIDS support groups, and help C.Q. call a friend to accompany her home this evening. She looks at you through her tears and states, "I can't believe it. J. is the only man I've had sex with since my divorce. He told me I had nothing to worry about. I can't believe he would do this to me."

3.   C.Q.'s statement is based on 3 assumptions: that J. is HIV-positive, that he intentionally withheld that information from her, and that he intentionally transmitted the HIV to her through unprotected sex. Based on your knowledge of HIV infection, how would you counsel C.Q.?

4. In addition to offering alternative explanations and exploring alternatives, what is your most important role at this time?

5. Identify 4 nursing diagnoses for C.Q.

6. C.Q. had a positive EIA test and is seropositive for HIV, why doesn't she have signs or symptoms of infection of AIDS?

7. What assessment findings would support a diagnoses of AIDS?

8. Why is it a good idea that someone C.Q. trusts escort her home this evening?

C.Q. gives you the name and phone number of a relative she wants you to call. You remain with her until she leaves with her relative.

9. Has C.Q.'s right to privacy been violated? Explain why or why not?

10. C.Q. returns to the office 4 days later to discuss her diagnosis. What issues will you discuss with her at this time?

11. Does C.Q. have a legal responsibility to inform J. of her HIV status?

Two weeks later C.Q. visits the office and asks to speak to you in private. She thanks you for talking to her the day she received the news of her diagnosis. She pulls a gun from her purse and states, "I was going to go out into the waiting room and blow J. away, because I thought he was cheating on me." She tells you that J. confessed to her he was afraid to tell her about his hemophilia because she might leave him. J. is HIV tested at regular intervals and his last HIV test, 6 months ago, had been negative. J. was retested and was positive for HIV. J.'s doctor discussed the possibility of transmission through recombinant factor VIII products. C.Q. tells you that they are going to get married and invites you to the wedding. She stops at the door and says, "At least we won't have to worry about 'safe sex' with each other!"

Case Study 3

K.D. is a 36-year-old gay professional man who has been HIV positive for 6 years. Until recently, he demonstrated no signs or symptoms of AIDS. The appearance of purplish spots on his neck and arms persuaded him to make an appointment with his physician. Upon arrival at the doctor's office, the nurse performed a brief assessment. His VS were 138/86, 100, 30, 100.8°F. K.D. stated that he had been feeling fatigued for several months and is experiencing occasional night sweats but he had been working long hours, was skipping meals, and had been particularly stressed over a project at work. K.D.'s physical was within normal limits except for his low-grade fever and skin lesions. The doctor ordered a CBC, lymphocyte studies, and a PPD. K.D. made an appointment to return in 5 days to discuss the results of his tests.

Over the next 2 weeks, K.D. developed a fever of 101°F, nonproductive cough, and increasing shortness of breath. At midnight he became acutely SOB, so his roommate, J.F., took K.D. to the ED where he was subsequently admitted to the hospital with probable *Pneumocystis carinii* pneumonia. Bronchoalveolar lavage examined under light microscopy confirmed the diagnosis. K.D.'s admission WBC and lymphocyte studies demonstrated a increased pattern of immunodeficiency from earlier studies. K.D. was placed on nasal oxygen, IV fluids, and IV trimethoprim/sulfamethazine (Septra).

1. What is *Pneumocystis carinii* pneumonia (PCP)?

2. What is the significance of the purplish spots over K.D.'s neck and arms?

3. Identify 4 nursing diagnoses for K.D.

4. What precautions will you need to use when caring for K.D.?

5. What will be the focus of your ongoing assessment (list 5)?

6. What major side effects of the drug Septra should you monitor K.D. for?

7. Compare and contrast HIV positive status with AIDS.

8. Why is K.D.'s development of PCP of particular importance in light of his HIV status?

9. K.D. has been seropositive for several years, yet has been asymptomatic for AIDS. What factors may have influenced K.D.'s development of pneumocystis?

K.D. is responding well to treatment and plans are being made for discharge. He will be started on AZT therapy and inhaled pentamidine, and followed on an outpatient basis.

10. K.D. was taught about disease transmission and safe sex, as well as encouraged to maintain good exercise, rest, and dietary habits when he was diagnosed as HIV positive. Give at least 4 additional topics that should be discussed with K.D. before he goes home.

11. What laboratory data will most likely be monitored on K.D. in the future?

12. List at least 5 other opportunistic infections that K.D. is at risk for developing.

Case Study 4

Name: _____ Class/Group: _____ Date: _____

Instructions: All questions apply to this case study. Your response should be brief and to the point. Adequate space has been provided for answers. When asked to provide several answers, they should be listed in order of priority or significance. Do not assume information that is not provided. Please print or write legibly.

J.P., a 56-year-old man, developed a severe viral infection and suffered fatigue, fever, and myalgia. Although he recovered from the acute episode, J.P. never quite regained normal activity level. Six months later, J.P. continued to find it difficult to work a 10-hour day as a brick mason so he returned to his physician. Diagnostic studies revealed CHF r/t postviral cardiomyopathy. Following medical management with digoxin (Lanoxin) and furosemide (Lasix), his condition stabilized and he returned to work, but his attendance was erratic. J.P.'s condition gradually deteriorated, and he was readmitted to the hospital 16 months later with complaints of dyspnea with minimal exertion, fatigue, orthopnea, chest pain, anorexia, and feelings of abdominal fullness. He had 1 + peripheral edema and was diaphoretic. Further studies revealed that J.P. had cardiac dilation, moderate to gross ventricular hypertrophy, and poor systolic ejection fraction, consistent with severe congestive cardiomyopathy. Because J.P.'s only other health problem is mild hypertension, heart transplant evaluation was recommended. J.P. and his wife discussed his prognosis and agreed to an evaluation for possible heart transplantation.

1. If J.P. is accepted for cardiac transplantation, what data will be collected in addition to his past medical history, current diagnostic findings, and cardiac evaluation?

2. What criteria for heart transplantation does J.P. meet that will make him eligible for cardiac transplantation?

3. Cite 5 contraindications for cardiac transplant.

4. J.P. is accepted for cardiac transplant and placed on the waiting list. What fears or concerns may J.P. experience during this waiting period?

J.P. received a phone call to report to the hospital immediately because a donor heart had become available.

5.   What compatibility tests are preformed to determine eligibility for transplantation and to ensure as close a match as possible?

6.   As the nurse on the transplant unit, how can you best help J.P. prepare for his heart transplant?

J.P.'s surgery and recovery were uncomplicated and he was sent home and referred to cardiac rehabilitation after adjustment of his immunosuppression therapy and appropriate teaching. J.P. was readmitted for low grade fever and dyspnea 6 weeks after surgery. Cardiac biopsies demonstrated moderate acute rejection.

7.   What is the etiology of acute rejection and how does it differ from chronic rejection?

8. The nurse can anticipate that prompt immunosuppressive therapy will be instituted using what drug? How does this drug alter the rejection process?

9. What is the most important nursing intervention for J.P. at this time and why?

J.P. responded positively to steroid therapy and was released to home after 5 days. J.P. was again admitted to the hospital with renewed complaints of dyspnea, low-grade fever, and ankle swelling 7 months later. Both J.P. and his wife are anxious and fearful.

10. Explain what may be happening to J.P. physiologically.

11. How will treatment for this episode of graft rejection differ from treatment for his earlier episode of rejection?

12. J.P.'s prognosis for the future will depend on what factors?

Case Study 5

Name: _____ *Class/Group:* _____ *Date:* _____

Instructions: All questions apply to this case study. Your response should be brief and to the point. Adequate space has been provided for answers. When asked to provide several answers, they should be listed in order of priority or significance. Do not assume information that is not provided. Please print or write legibly.

W.V. is a 47-year-old man who lives with his wife and 2 teen-aged sons. W.V. developed chronic renal failure 12 years ago after acute renal failure due to phenacetin use. W.V. has taken phenacetin since his early 20s for migraine headaches. Large doses of phenacetin over the years can cause analgesic-induced nephropathy. This drug was subsequently removed from the market. W.V. was initially placed on hemodialysis but was switched to peritoneal dialysis so he could remain employed as an auto mechanic. Three months ago W.V. received a cadaveric transplant, or cadaver kidney. He recovered without complications and his serum laboratory values returned to normal. He was placed on immunosuppressive therapy, including cyclosporine (Sandimmune), and prednisone (Orasone) and was discharged to home. W.V. returned to work 3 weeks later.

Today W.V. reported to his physician for routine follow-up. His VS are 148/92, 88, 24, 99.2°F. His lab data revealed a serum creatinine 1.2 mg/dl and BUN 22 mg/dl, with normal serum electrolytes. W.V. has gained 5 pounds since discharge from the hospital.

1. What histocompatibility studies are generally performed before renal transplant and why are they important?

2. By what criteria was W.V. considered a good candidate for renal transplantation?

3. If W.V.'s kidney is producing sufficient urine and he is feeling well, why is it necessary to monitor his laboratory data?

4. What is the possible significance of W.V.'s current blood pressure?

5. How does the drug cyclosporine (Sandimmune) protect W.V.'s kidney from rejection, and what are the most important side effects of this drug that W.V. must be taught to monitor?

6. Because of the side effects of cyclosporine, how will W.V. know if he is experiencing organ rejection?

7. If W.V. begins to reject his kidney, how would the rejection be classified, and what signs and symptoms would most likely be present?

8. Identify at least 4 ways that W.V. might experience difficulty adjusting to his organ transplant.

9. How can you best support W.V. and his family?

10. Why is it necessary for W.V. to be concerned about infection?

Case Study 6

Name: _____ Class/Group: _____ Date: _____

Instructions: All questions apply to this case study. Your response should be brief and to the point. Adequate space has been provided for answers. When asked to provide several answers, they should be listed in order of priority or significance. Do not assume information that is not provided. Please print or write legibly.

D.C. is a 32-year-old white clerical worker who lives with his 76-year-old grandmother, his primary caregiver. He was diagnosed as being HIV positive 3 months ago and has been under close outpatient medical supervision for the past 3 weeks because of persistent fever, pulmonary infiltrates, and nonspecific flu like symptoms. He is admitted to your nursing unit for fever, chills, sweats, myalgias, malaise, chest pain, dry nonproductive cough, axillary adenopathy, nausea, vomiting, and severe diarrhea. Admission VS are 108/84, 104, 30, 103.5°F. Following aggressive diagnostic workup, D.C. was diagnosed with AIDS complicated by *Pneumocystis carinii* pneumonia, cryptosporidiosis, oral candidiasis, and cytomegalovirus (CMV) infection.

Today is D.C.'s third day postadmission to the hospital. He remains acutely ill; however, his hydration status has improved and he is experiencing fewer than 8 diarrhea stools per day. He is not yet able to keep food or fluids down; therefore, TPN is being considered. D.C. complains of headache, nausea, continued fatigue, and muscle soreness. He is able to ambulate to the bathroom with assistance.

1. Why was D.C. diagnosed as having AIDS rather than complicated HIV infection?

2. Considering D.C.'s AIDS status, what findings are likely to be present when you receive the results of his lymphocyte studies?

3. Provide a possible explanation for D.C.'s rapid conversion from HIV positive to AIDS.

4. As D.C.'s nurse, list at least 2 observations you would monitor in relation to each of the following infections: cryptosporidiosis, candidiasis, and CMV.

5. Given the above possible problems that D.C. could encounter, which of the following nursing orders would be appropriate? Label each with "A" for appropriate or "I" for inappropriate and correct the inappropriate orders.
    ___ Monitor VS every 12 hours.

    ___ Assist with ADL as needed.

    ___ Keep perineal area clean and dry; use protective skin cream.

    ___ Regular diet.

    ___ Monitor lungs, skin, abdomen, and urine output once per shift.

    ___ Maintain complete bed rest.

    ___ Use toothettes or soft-bristled brush for oral hygiene.

    ___ Exclude diarrhea stool from I&O measurements.

    ___ Monitor IV site for signs of inflammation; change site if red or swollen.

6. D.C. is restless at times because of his muscle soreness. Upon entering his room you note that he has pulled out his peripheral IV and is bleeding. How should you respond?

7. Cite at least 5 findings that would indicate D.C.'s condition is stabilizing or improving.

8. What assessment findings would the physician take into consideration when making the decision to place D.C. on TPN?

9. Given that D.C.'s grandmother is his primary caregiver, discuss the implications of D.C.'s diagnosis of AIDS.

10. Would D.C. require additional teaching regarding his ability to transmit HIV now that he has AIDS?

11. D.C. begins to slowly respond to treatment, and discharge plans are begun. Cite at least 3 ways that D.C.'s post-AIDS care will differ from his pre-AIDS care.

12. How does AZT work to control progression of HIV? Can you confirm or refute this explanation?

Case Study 7

Name: _____ Class/Group: _____ Date: _____

Instructions: All questions apply to this case study. Your response should be brief and to the point. Adequate space has been provided for answers. When asked to provide several answers, they should be listed in order of priority or significance. Do not assume information that is not provided. Please print or write legibly.

D.W. is a 23-year-old married woman with 3 children under the age of 5. She presented to her physician 2 years ago with vague complaints of intermittent fatigue, joint pain, and low-grade fever. Her physician noted small patchy areas of vitiligo and a scaly rash across her nose, cheeks, back, and chest at that time. Laboratory studies revealed that D.W. had a positive antinuclear antibody titer, positive LE (lupus erythematosus) cell prep, elevated C-reactive protein and ESR (erythrocytesedimentation rate), and decreased C3 and C4 serum complement. Joint x-rays demonstrated joint swelling without joint erosion. D.W. was subsequently diagnosed with systemic lupus erythematosus. She was initially treated with sulindac (Clinopri) 200 mg PO bid and prednisone (Deltasone) 20 mg PO qd, bed rest, ice packs, and aspirin to control discomfort. She was counseled regarding her condition, advised to balance rest and activity, eat a well-balanced diet, use strategies to reduce stress, and avoid direct sunlight. D.W. responded well to treatment and was eventually told she could report for follow-up every 6 months unless her symptoms became acute. D.W. resumed her job in environmental services at a large geriatric facility.

1. What is the significance of each of D.W.'s laboratory findings?

2. How does cutaneous lupus erythematosus differ from systemic lupus?

3. What priority problems need to be addressed with D.W.?

Eighteen months after diagnosis, D.W. sought out her physician because of puffy hands and feet and increased fatigue. D.W. reported that she had been working longer hours because of the absence of 2 of her fellow workers. Diagnostic evaluation revealed that her BUN and serum creatinine were slightly elevated, and that she had 2+ protein and 1+ RBC in her urine.

4.   Of what significance are these findings, and what is the relationship of such findings to D.W.'s diagnosis of lupus erythematosus?

5.   How will D.W.'s treatment and nursing plan likely change?

D.W. was seen in the immunology clinic twice monthly during the next 3 months. Although her condition did not worsen, her BUN and serum creatinine remained elevated. While at work one afternoon, D.W. began to feel dizzy and developed a severe headache. She reported to her supervisor who had her lie down. When D.W. started to become disoriented, her supervisor called 911 and had D.W. taken to the hospital. D.W. was admitted for probable lupus cerebritis related to acute exacerbation of her disease.

6.   What preventive measures should be instituted to protect D.W. at this time?

7.   What additional problems indicative of CNS involvement related to systemic lupus should D.W. be assessed for?

D.W. is again placed on IV methylprednisolone and started on plasmapheresis.

8.   What major complications associated with immunosuppression therapy will D.W. have to be monitored for?

9.   What does plasmapheresis do, and why might it reduce the signs and symptoms associated with systemic lupus?

10. What data would support the assumption that D.W.'s condition is stabilizing?

11. Identify at least 4 topics that D.W. must be taught before she is discharged that may help her lead as normal a life as possible.

12. You note that D.W.'s husband is visiting her this afternoon. You enter the room to ask if they have any questions. D.W.'s husband states, "I have tried to tell her that she cannot go back to work. Sure we need the money but the kids and I need her more. I'm afraid that this lupus has weakened her whole body and it will kill her if she goes back to work. Is that right?" How would you respond to his concerns?

CHAPTER 9. ONCOLOGIC/HEMATOLOGIC DISORDERS

Case Study 1

Name: _____ Class/Group: _____ Date: _____

Instructions: All questions apply to this case study. Your response should be brief and to the point. Adequate space has been provided for answers. When asked to provide several answers, they should be listed in order of priority or significance. Do not assume information that is not provided. Please print or write legibly.

B.B., a 53-year-old divorced professional woman, was diagnosed with stage T1 N0 infiltrating ductal breast cancer based on a lumpectomy and axillary lymph node dissection over a year ago. After her radiation therapy (daily treatments for 6 weeks) was completed, she was placed on tamoxifen for an indefinite period. She has been coming to the clinic every 3 months for her checkup. In addition to working at the clinic, you are a volunteer consultant to the Encore-YWCA support group for women who have had breast cancer that B.B. attends regularly. The group invited you to present "Breast Cancer: Prevention, Screening, and Detection Guidelines" at their next meeting.

1. Describe estrogen replacement therapy (ERT) and the relationship to breast cancer.

2. What is tamoxifen? Why are women placed on long-term tamoxifen therapy as a treatment for breast cancer?

3. What is an axillary lymph node dissection? Why did B.B. have an axillary lymph node dissection with her lumpectomy?

4. B.B. was diagnosed with stage T1 N0 breast cancer. What does that mean?

5. What risk factors for breast cancer will you include in your group presentation?
    •   Risk factors include:

6. What will you teach them about early detection of breast cancer?

7. What educational equipment can help women learn how to correctly perform BSE and how to detect lumps?

8. Describe the technique for performing BSE correctly.

9. One of the women in the group shows you how the arm on the side with the breast cancer is more swollen than the other arm. She said she is having a lot of trouble with this. What do you think is happening? How will you explain this to her? What will you advise her?

10. B.B. raises her hand and tells you she heard she should never have her blood pressure taken in her affected arm (the arm on the side of the breast cancer). You remember you told her this in the office but realize she was probably too anxious or tired to remember what you said. What will you advise her and the other women present?

11. What are some other things breast cancer survivors can do to manage or prevent lymphedema (list 4)?

Case Study 2

Name: _____ Class/Group: _____ Date: _____

Instructions: All questions apply to this case study. Your response should be brief and to the point. Adequate space has been provided for answers. When asked to provide several answers, they should be listed in order of priority or significance. Do not assume information that is not provided. Please print or write legibly.

V.M. is a 39-year-old black man who has sickle cell disease (SCD) marked by frequent episodes of severe pain. His anemia has been managed with multiple transfusions, and he shows signs of chronic renal failure. He is a nonsmoker, nondrinker, and is on Social Security disability. His regular medications are pentoxifylline (Trental), oxycodone/acetaminophen (Roxicet), and folic acid (Folvite). In hematology clinic this AM, V.M.'s Hgb measured 6.7 g/dl. He received 2 units PRC (packed red cells) over 3 hours and then went home. V.M. developed dyspnea and shortness of breath approximately 1 to 1½ hours later, and his wife called 911. The EMS (emergency medical system) crew initiated oxygen and transported V.M. to the ED.

1. What is sickle cell disease, and how is it related to race?

2. The stiff, sickled RBC tends to cause vascular occlusions with subsequent local infarction. As a rule, the spleen suffers so many vasoocclusive/infarction episodes that it is greatly reduced in size and is rendered nonfunctional by the time the individual is 6 years of age. What are the implications of having a nonfunctioning spleen?

3. Identify 2 mechanisms that contribute to anemia in patients with SCD.

4. On arrival to the ED, the physician asks V.M. if he is in pain and if he needs Demerol. V.M. answers "No" to both questions. Why did the physician ask these 2 questions?

5. V.M.'s ABGs on 9 L O_2/simple face mask are pH 7.34, PaO_2 74 mm Hg, $PaCO_2$ 33 mm Hg, HCO_3 18 mEq/L, BE -6. Is V.M. being adequately oxygenated, why or why not?

6. V.M. complains of being short of breath. Do you believe his low Hgb level is responsible for his complaints?

You perform a quick assessment and note a systolic murmur and crackles in V.M.'s bases bilaterally. VS are 176/102, 94, 28, 97°F (oral). As you start an IV, you draw blood for CBC, Chem 7, calcium, and phosphorous and send it for analysis.

7. Your assessment findings are consistent with fluid overload. What 4 findings led you to that conclusion?

8. What action would you expect the physician to take next and why?

The lab values return: Na 137 mEq/L, K 4.9 mEq/L, Cl 110 mEq/L, CO_2 16 mEq/L, BUN 27 mg/dl, creatinine 2.7 mg/dl, calcium 8.2 mg/dl, PO_4 4.7 mg/dl, WBC 4.3 mm^3, Hgb 7.8 g/dl, Hct 20.9%, platelets 208 mm^3.

9. What is the significance of the lab results and why?

The physician prescribes furosemide (Lasix) 20 mg IVP now, methylprednisolone (Solu-Medrol) 125 mg IVP, and ceftriaxone (Rocephin) 1 g IVPB after the Lasix.

10. Explain the significance of using each of these drugs.

11. Why is it difficult to cross-match blood to transfuse V.M.?

As V.M.'s SOB is relieved, he shakes the physician's hand and thanks him for asking about the presence of pain and the need for pain medication. V.M. states, "One of my biggest fears is that I'll come here in crisis and the doctor won't treat my pain aggressively enough. I don't want to be labeled as a drug seeker or an emergency room abuser."

12. Why would V.M. be concerned about obtaining adequate pain control in the ED?

V.M. voids 1900 ml within 2 hours of the Lasix administration. On repeat assessment, the systolic murmur is audible, but all lung fields are clear. Repeat VS are 160/94, 82, 20, 98°F (oral). V.M. is discharged to home on his previous medications.

13. What issues would you address with V.M. before he is discharged?

Case Study 3

Name: _____ Class/Group: _____ Date: _____

Instructions: All questions apply to this case study. Your response should be brief and to the point. Adequate space has been provided for answers. When asked to provide several answers, they should be listed in order of priority or significance. Do not assume information that is not provided. Please print or write legibly.

D.M. is a married, 36-year-old woman with 4 children who works part-time as a clerk. She is 68 in tall and weighs 135 lb. She has insurance through her husband's employer. She has never smoked and has an occasional social drink. She has PMH of plastic surgery for breast implants in August of last year. When she returned for her breast implant check-up 10 months later, a lump was discovered in her R breast. When a biopsy indicated the lump was malignant, she elected to have a lumpectomy and axillary lymph node dissection. Her CT scan and bone scans were negative. She was referred to the group oncology clinic where you are a staff nurse to receive chemotherapy. After she completes chemotherapy, she is scheduled to receive radiation therapy. Admitting diagnosis: infiltrating ductal carcinoma, stage T2 N1 M0, premenopausal, estrogen receptor-positive.

1. Explain the TNM method of staging malignancies.

2. D.M. wants you to explain exactly what stage T2 N1 M0 means. What will you tell her?

3. She asks you to explain what her chances of survival are. How will you explain this to her?

4. D.M. will be receiving 6 cycles of combination chemotherapy, consisting of doxirubicin (Adriamycin), cyclophosphamide (Cytoxan), and 5-fluorouracil (5-FU). What are the major side effects you want to prepare her for?

5.   What is a major complication in patients receiving a high amount of Adriamycin?

6.   Explain to D.M. in lay terms what she needs to know about immunosuppression.

D.M. completes her chemotherapy. She lost most of her hair and has been wearing a scarf but now her hair is beginning to grow back. She is being transferred to the radiation therapy department for treatment and is scheduled to begin radiation therapy.

7.   What is hair loss called? Which drug was primarily responsible for the hair loss?

You perform an admission assessment. Findings are: Wt. 148 lb. VS 104/70, 80, 20, 98.0°F (oral). Cardiovascular: S1 S2 without murmurs or rubs. Respiratory: clear to auscultation throughout. Neuromuscular/skeletal: negative, patient c/o of fatigue, no c/o bone pain. GI: without hepatosplenomegaly or masses. GU: negative. Integumentary/oral: hair growth ¼" over entire head, oral mucosa reddened and patient c/o soreness. Lymph node: no palpable adenopathy in the cervical, supraclavicular, axillary, or inguinal nodes.

8.   What areas of the above assessment concern you? Explain.

D.M. received 6 weeks of daily (weekdays) radiation therapy treatments with a total dose of 6400 cGy. She had a terrible time with fatigue, and at one time, told you, "When I lie down, I can't be enough of the bed!" You helped her develop an activity-rest plan and supported her in obtaining outside help with housework. At her last visit, she tells you, "Now I hope I can see my kids grow up." She is scheduled to return to the oncologist every 3 months for follow-up care and monitoring.

9. D.M. comes to her scheduled follow-up appointment. She appears very anxious. When questioned she tells you, "I've been worried about my daughters. What if they get breast cancer? What can I do to help them?" What is your response?

10. You ask her if she has other questions. She tells you she is worried about the breast cancer coming back and wants to know if she would have to go through the chemotherapy and radiation therapy all over again. What can you do, and what will you tell her?

D.M. seemed to do fine for a while. On her 9-month follow-up visit, she tells you she has been having headaches for the past few weeks. Her MRI indicates she has metastases to the brain. She underwent a bone marrow transplant; unfortunately, it failed to stop her cancer. She died at the age of 38, leaving behind 4 children aged 4 through 14.

Case Study 4

Name: _____ Class/Group: _____ Date: _____

Instructions: All questions apply to this case study. Your response should be brief and to the point. Adequate space has been provided for answers. When asked to provide several answers, they should be listed in order of priority or significance. Do not assume information that is not provided. Please print or write legibly.

A.V. is a 37-year-old, married housewife, with a 35 pack/year history of smoking. She says she "just can't quit." She denies ETOH use. Ht 67" Wt 115 lb. Her PMH includes C-sections for all 3 children ages 6, 14, and 18. She does not have insurance. She noticed a "canker sore" on the anterior lateral aspect of her L tongue several months ago. Over time, she developed a sore throat and ear pain. The family nurse practitioner at the low-income clinic sent her to a specialist who performed a biopsy of her anterior tongue. The diagnosis was squamous cell carcinoma—poorly differentiated—T2 N0. Before her surgery she had complete Panorex views of her mandible; fluoride trays were made followed by a partial glossectomy and excision of the floor of her mouth. Three weeks after surgery, multiple teeth are scheduled to be extracted. Afterward, she will be scheduled for 8 weeks of radiation therapy in your outpatient clinic.

1. Describe the rationale for this prophylactic treatment: teeth extraction, Panorex views, fluoride trays.

2. Identify and describe preop nursing care for partial glossectomy.

3. Identify and describe potential postop care for partial glossectomy.

4. Identify and describe potential postop complications resulting from a partial glossectomy. Plan appropriate nursing interventions and patient teaching strategies to manage these complications.

5. When she returns for her first postop visit to your clinic, she appears to be quite distressed to hear about the radiation therapy. Although she still has considerable trouble speaking, she explains she really didn't think much about it before surgery. She seems quite embarrassed as she tells you her family has no insurance, and they were barely making it earlier. Now she says she is getting "nasty letters" from the hospital demanding payment. What can you do?

6. As she sits by you, she keeps her hand over her mouth and jaw. She is wearing her hair so if hangs down over her face. Her jaw and neck still are swollen from the surgery and tooth extraction. She avoids eye contact with you. How will you respond?

Case Study 5

Name: _____ Class/Group: _____ Date: _____

Instructions: All questions apply to this case study. Your response should be brief and to the point. Adequate space has been provided for answers. When asked to provide several answers, they should be listed in order of priority or significance. Do not assume information that is not provided. Please print or write legibly.

A.T. is a 21-year-old college student. He works part-time as a manual laborer, uses a half can/week of smokeless tobacco, and drinks a 6 pack of beer/week. A year ago in September, he discovered a small, painless lump in his lower L neck. Over the quarter, he experienced increasing fatigue and a 10-lb weight loss that he attributed to "working and studying too hard." In the spring, he saw a nurse practitioner at the student health center who immediately referred him to an oncologist. A lymph node biopsy revealed Hodgkin's disease. The CT scan of the chest, abdomen, and pelvis; gallium scan; and bone scan all came back negative. A staging laparotomy was conducted a month later to confirm the diagnosis. His diagnosis was Hodgkin's disease stage IA mixed cellularity. You are a staff nurse in the outpatient oncology services when A.T. comes in.

1. A.T. wants to know what Hodgkin's disease is and how he "caught" it. What will you tell him?

2. A.T. wants to know what "stage IA" means; he also wants to know the significance of the test results. What are you going to tell him?

A few days later, you see A.T. in the oncologist's office during his appointment to discuss the treatment regimen for radiation therapy. His prescribed radiation treatment regimen (outpatient) includes Monday through Friday with treatments scheduled for approximately 6 to 10 weeks. Admission assessment findings on his first visit to the outpatient oncology clinic at the end of January are Wt 183 lb, Ht 78 in. VS 124/66, 60, 16, 98.0°F (oral). Cardiovascular: heart rate regular. Respiratory: clear to auscultation. Neuromuscular/skeletal, GI, and GU: negative. Integumentary/oral: incision from staging laparotomy well-approximated without erythema, edema, pain, or drainage. Incision from lymph node dissection healing well, oral mucosa pink and moist, no palpable adenopathy.

3. What abnormal assessment findings do you find in the above information?

4. A.T. jokes with you that he's going to get nuked and "glow." What information would you include in your teaching for someone like A.T. to prepare her/him for radiation treatments?

5. You have developed a good relationship with A.T. during the multiple visits required for his radiation therapy. He shares some futuristic goals and says, "What are the chances that I will beat this cancer?" Respond to A.T.'s request.

Other kinds of cancer may occur many years later as a result of the toxic effects of earlier treatment. This is one reason why cancer specialists are reluctant to use the word "cured."

6. What other issues of survivorship may affect patients like A.T. (e.g., insurance, employability)?

7. How and what are you going to counsel and teach A.J. about potential sterility/infertility side effects of treatment?

8. Six weeks into therapy, A.T. drags himself into the clinic one Friday, drops into a chair, and wearily states, "I'm quitting. If this is what life is like, it's not worth living." How would you respond to him?

9. When A.T. checked in this week, he weighed 177 lb. When you express concern, he tells you he just doesn't have any appetite. How are you going to respond? List at least 4 interventions.

10. At his final appointment, A.T.'s laboratory values are WBC 3.3 mm^3, Hgb 14 g/dl, Hct 41%, and platelets 369 mm^3. His VS are 120/76, 84, 20, 98.0°F(oral). Wt 175 lb. Do any of these values concern you? Explain.

A.T. was discharged from radiation and scheduled to see an oncologist every 3 months for follow-up care.

Case Study 6

C.W. is a 42-year-old, divorced woman with adenocarcinoma (cancer) of the lung with
metastasis (spread) to the brain and liver. She is the single parent of a 17-year-old son, has
experienced episodic health care, is currently unemployed because of poor health, and has
no health insurance. She has smoked 1 to 2 packs/day for 20 years. PMH includes
cholecystectomy, hysterectomy, and breast augmentation. In May of last year, she
developed scapular and arm pain in her right side, was diagnosed with adenocarcinoma of
the lung, and underwent a wedge resection of the upper right lobe of the lung. Because
she had no insurance, she did not receive follow-up care (e.g., radiation therapy and/or
chemotherapy).

C.W. developed pain in her right temple 48 hours ago and was seen in the ED, where she
was given cephradine (Velosef). C.W. had a seizure 24 hours later, was transported to the
ED, and was diagnosed as having an allergic reaction to the Velosef. She was instructed to
call her family doctor. C.W.'s doctor was unavailable for 48 hours. After suffering a tonic-
clonic (grand mal) seizure at home, she was admitted to a rural hospital. A CT scan
revealed a large mass in the right frontal area of her brain. Dexamethasone (Decadron) was
given IV, and an oncologist in the metropolitan area was consulted. C.W. was transferred
to your oncology unit postseizure with slight slurred speech and intermittent bone pain.
She has lost 22 lb. in the past year. She is receiving acetaminophen/hydrocodone (Lortab)
1-2 5 mg tabs every 3 to 4 hours, as needed. C.W.'s record lists codeine and milk
allergies.

1.   Identify the usual location, growth rate, and likelihood of metastasis of
     adenocarcinoma of the lung.

2.   Is the presence of bone pain and weight loss significant?

3.   What tests are likely to be performed to determine if C.W.'s adenocarcinoma has
     metastasized?

4. The tests are performed, and C.W. is diagnosed with adenocarcinoma of the lung with metastasis to lymph nodes, liver, and brain. She is scheduled to receive 10 radiation therapy treatments to the whole brain (3 as an inpatient, 7 as an outpatient). Identify 5 needs that you will address with C.W. and her son.

After her third radiation treatment, C.W. is discharged on the following medications: dexamethasone (Decadron) 4 mg PO q8h; propoxyphene/acetaminophen (Darvocet-N) 100 mg PO q4h PRN; prochloperazine maleate (Compazine Spansule) 15 mg PO q12h PRN; temazepam (Restoril) 30 mg PO q hs PRN.

5. What is the rationale for C.W. receiving each medication?

Two months posthospital discharge and follow-up therapy, C.W. continues to have increasing symptoms of pain, anorexia, weight loss, edema in extremities, and insomnia. Her son accompanied her to the physician's office. While his mother is having her blood drawn, he asks the nurse what is going to happen to his mother.

6. How would you respond to him?

7. He asks what he can do to help his mother. What information could you give him?
   • Things he can do to help are:

8.   As C.W.'s disease progresses, what signs and symptoms can be anticipated, and what kind of relief can be provided?

9.   C.W.'s son says he's never been around someone who is dying before. He expresses fear he won't know what to do. How can you help him?

Case Study 7

Name: _____ Class/Group: _____ Date: _____

Instructions: All questions apply to this case study. Your response should be brief and to the point. Adequate space has been provided for answers. When asked to provide several answers, they should be listed in order of priority or significance. Do not assume information that is not provided. Please print or write legibly.

D.L., a 21-year-old, single, plumber's assistant developed low back pain "from a work injury" 2 weeks ago. He had no PMH and is a nonsmoker, nondrinker. He was instructed to take diclofenac (Cataflam) 50 mg PO tid for 6 doses and cyclobenzaprine (Flexeril) 10 mg PO tid for 6 doses. Within 2 to 3 days, he developed a fever (101.6°F, oral), and a rash developed over his entire body. He showed dramatic bruising; he also developed a decreased appetite and a sore mouth. He was taken to the ER at a rural hospital when he started vomiting blood. His labs were WBC 31.7 mm^3, Hgb 10.1 g/dl, Hct 29%, and platelets 16 mm^3. Arrangements were made to transfer him to the regional medical center, where you work on the heme/onc unit, to see an oncologist for a workup and to be admitted to the hospital for therapy. A bone marrow biopsy confirmed the diagnosis of acute lymphoblastic leukemia.

1. What is acute lymphoblastic leukemia (ALL), and what are other names for this same condition?

2. You are the leukemia support and education group leader for your hospital. Patients attending your sessions have acute/chronic lymphocytic leukemia, acute/chronic myelogenous leukemia, myelodysplastic syndrome, and multiple myeloma. Your topic for discussion today is the etiology of the hematologic diseases for the previously stated diseases. D.L.'s older brother, T.L., is a nursing student and he wants to know how many kinds of leukemia there are, and if they are caused by the same thing. List the related diseases in the leukemia family and what is thought to cause each.

3. D.L. asks you what the chances are for someone, like himself, with ALL. What can you tell him?

D.L. is scheduled to receive the initial *induction* combination chemotherapy by IV and IT (intrathecal) routes. He will be receiving doxorubicin (Adriamycin), vincristine and cyclophosphamide (Cytoxan) IVP, methotrexate IT, and prednisone PO. He will be hospitalized about 3 weeks. He will be scheduled for intense *consolidation* courses, and then *maintenance* therapy for 1 year. The induction and consolidation courses are intense drug therapies, requiring multiple blood product infusions and antibiotic therapy to aid recovery. Because of his recent employment and projected required course of therapy, he will be unable to work and will probably lose his insurance.

D.L.'s admission assessments are: VS 140/74, 90, 24, 103.3°F (oral); Wt 150 lb; cardiovascular: normal sinus rhythm, no S_3, S_4 rubs, or murmurs, all peripheral pulses present; respiratory: clear to auscultation; neuromuscular/skeletal: grossly intact; motor and sensory exam normal; GI: spleen about 5 fingerbreadths below the right costal margin-tender, liver is not enlarged, no ascites or intraabdominal mass or CVA tenderness; GU: rectal not done; integumentary/oral: HEENT, nomocephalic, pupils level, round, reactive to light in accommodation, no sclera icterus, conjunctivas very pale, fundoscopic exam is benign; oropharynx has some gingival lesions, mucous membranes are moist and pale; tympanic membranes are normal; neck: supple, trachea midline, thyroid normal, no murmurs or JVD distention. To facilitate D.L.'s chemotherapy and blood product infusion, a triple-lumen subclavian catheter is inserted.

4. Describe potential effects the acute leukemia, treatment, and rehabilitation have on the socioeconomic status and family relationships of people like D.L.

5. During the next 14 days, D.L. receives irradiated platelets and leukoreduced, irradiated RBCs. What is the rationale for using irradiated, leukoreduced blood products? Describe the nursing administration/monitoring procedure for these products.

6. D.L. will continue to receive intense combination chemotherapy for several more weeks. Because of limited finances, his hospitalization stay will be cut short. What are the major self-care management issues for home care that need to be reinforced?

7. D.L. is going to be staying with his parents. T.L. has promised to help with D.L.'s care. In addition, a home care nurse will visit him twice weekly. You are going to teach D.L. and his brother, T.L., to care for and use his triple-lumen subclavian catheter. What will you tell them?

Before he leaves, T.L. says, "You know, I've been studying about some of this stuff in my med/surg class, but I had no idea how bad it feels to go through this. I hope this makes me a better, more sensitive nurse."

Case Study 8

Name: _____ Class/Group: _____ Date: _____

Instructions: All questions apply to this case study. Your response should be brief and to the point. Adequate space has been provided for answers. When asked to provide several answers, they should be listed in order of priority or significance. Do not assume information that is not provided. Please print or write legibly.

C.P. is a 61-year-old married farmer, with a PMH of hernia surgery in 1955 and prostate surgery in 1969 for BPH (benign prostatic hypertrophy). C.P. does not drink but he has smoked for 40 years; the past 3 years he has smoked 2 to 3 packs/day. He has no known allergies. Six months ago, C.P. visited the local rural health clinic with c/o progressive cough and chest congestion. Despite a week of antibiotic therapy, C.P. continued to worsen; he experienced progressive dyspnea, productive cough, and began to have night sweats. C.P. refused to be admitted to the hospital ("There's no one to look after the cows") but agreed to go for a CXR. The radiologist read C.P.'s CXR as left hilar lung mass—probable lung cancer. C.P. was scheduled for a diagnostic fiberoptic bronchoscopy with endobronchial lung biopsy as an outpatient to confirm the diagnosis.

1. What is fiberoptic bronchoscopy? What information will a fiberoptic bronchoscopy with endobronchial lung biopsy provide?

2. As the nurse who works with the pulmonologist, it is your responsibility to prepare C.P. for the fiberoptic bronchoscopy procedure. What would you include in your teaching plan?

3. What will be your responsibility during and immediately after the bronchoscopy?

4. C.P. tolerates the procedure well. He returns to the office in 4 days to learn the results of his test. The pulmonologist tells C.P. and his wife that he has oat cell lung cancer and explains that it is a very fast-growing cancer that has no cure. This kind of lung cancer is directly related to C.P.'s history of smoking. What is your role at this time?

C.P. is scheduled to begin combination chemotherapy with cisplatin (Platinol) and etoposide (VePesid). He plans to continue to work the farm as long as possible; his brother-in-law has promised to help him.

5. How would you explain combination chemotherapy and how it works to C.P. and his wife?

6. C.P.'s wife tells you she's heard that chemotherapy makes you really sick. How would you explain chemotherapy side effects?

7. What are the most common side effects of cisplatin and VePesid?

8. Based on your knowledge of the most common side effects, what interventions should be incorporated into his plan of care?

9. C.P. needs to have a working understanding of how to balance his treatments with his work. You sit down with C.P. to plan a daily work/activity/rest schedule to accommodate his treatments and side effects. What concepts would you emphasize?

10. C.P. receives cisplatin 60 mg in 100 ml NS IV over 1 to 2 hours daily, the first 3 days of each month for 6 months, and VePesid 200 mg in 250 ml NS IV over 1 to 2 hours daily, the first 3 days of each month for 6 months. What is the nadir for each drug and what implications does the nadir have for C.P.?

A month later, when C.P. returns for his second round of chemotherapy, he c/o SOB, chest tightness, and palpitations. He looks exhausted. ECG and CXR reveal atrial fibrillation and LLL pneumonia with L pleural effusion. C.P. is admitted to the hospital with the following laboratory values: WBC 2.5 mm^3, RBC 5.6 mm^3, Hgb 17.7 g/dl, Hct 51.7%, platelets 252.0 mm^3, PT 12.1 sec, PTT 29.7 sec, Na 131 mEq/L, K 4.2 mEq/L, Cl 90 mEq/L, CO$_2$ 25 mEq/L, BUN 13 mg/dl, creatinine 0.8 mg/dl, glucose 175 mg/dl.

11. What do these lab values indicate?

12. The pulmonologist performs a thoracentesis and prescribes cefotaximine (Claforan) 1 g IV and q8h erythromycin (Erythrocin) 500 mg IV q6h. What factor in C.P.'s background will complicate his diagnosis of pneumonia?

13. C.P.'s condition continues to deteriorate. He tells you he doesn't want to live like this, but the doctor wants to continue with aggressive therapy. Discuss the pros and cons of continued therapy.

C.P. was given the second round of chemotherapy and was discharged to home. He never returned to the hospital for further treatment. He died 2 weeks later.

Case Study 9

You are caring for J.B., a 56-year-old woman with colon cancer. PMH includes colon resection followed by combined chemotherapy approximately 18 months ago; recently diagnosed with recurrence of colon cancer and chemotherapy was administered for 5 of the 8 scheduled cycles; previous significant weight loss (current Ht 67", Wt 105 lb); 50 pack/year (2 PPD x 25 yrs) smoking history. J.B. was admitted for acute nausea, vomiting, and dehydration. She is nutritionally depleted. Her physician determines that diagnostic evaluation requires exploratory laparotomy. VS 150/90, 124, 26, 100°F.

1. What are the major risks and potential complications for J.B.?

2. The physician performs an exploratory laparotomy for lysis of adhesions, small bowel resection, colectomy, and colostomy with Hartman's pouch. After surgery, J.B. is admitted to the SICU with a large abdominal dressing. You roll J.B. side-to-side to remove the soiled surgical linen, and the dressing becomes saturated with a large amount of serosanguinous drainage. Would the drainage be expected after abdominal surgery?

3. Traditionally, the physician performs the first dressing change. Why is this done?

4. The physician removes the surgical dressing. The wound edges are well approximated, the suture line is edematous, the staples are intact, the transverse colostomy rosebud looks pink in the middle and dark around the edges, and there is a Penrose drain in the RMQ. Do any of these findings concern you and why?

The physician prescribes the following TPN orders: amino acids 10% - 100 ml; dextrose 70% 1000 ml; water for injection 1000 ml; sodium acetate 20 mEq; sodium phosphate 20 mEq; potassium acetate 20 mEq; KCl 90 mEq; calcium gluconate 20 mEq; magnesium sulfate 10 mEq; regular insulin 10 units; multivitamins 1 amp; heparin 1200 units. Infuse 3000 ml volume over 24h daily.

5. What nursing management activities should you provide to minimize the potential side effects for J.B.?

6. The TPN infusion is complete, the alarm is sounding, and the pharmacy has not delivered the next bottle of TPN. What action should you take and why?

7. You explain to J.B. that she needs to dangle at the side of the bed for a few minutes, then get out of bed and sit in the chair. As J.B. attempts to stand at the bedside, the oxygen tubing pulls her head backward. You remove the oxygen while assisting J.B. to be seated in the chair, then replace the nasal cannula. What are the implications of your action?

8. Within minutes of sitting in the chair, you note that J.B. is becoming increasingly pale and diaphoretic. Her pulse is rapid and irregular and she c/o being nauseated and dizzy. What actions should you take next?

9. J.B. looks at you and tells you that she knows she is never going to leave the hospital alive. She says she has a lot of regrets. She confides that she used to drink a lot and wasn't a good mother to her 3 children; her son hasn't spoken to her in 15 years. How should you respond?

CHAPTER 10. MULTIPLE SYSTEM DISORDERS

Case Study 1

Name: _____ _____ *Class/Group:* _____ *Date:* _____

Instructions: All questions apply to this case study. Your response should be brief and to the point. Adequate space has been provided for answers. When asked to provide several answers, they should be listed in order of priority or significance. Do not assume information that is not provided. Please print or write legibly.

You are working the day shift on the medical-surgical unit in a small, rural community hospital. Your assignment includes an 18-year-old woman, A.N., admitted at night. She was burned in a house fire. She sustained 30% body surface and partial-thickness burns on her legs and back.

1. A.N. is undergoing burn fluid resuscitation using the standard Baxter (Parkland) formula. She was burned at 0200 and admitted at 0400. She weighs 110 pounds. Calculate her fluid requirements, and specify how much will be given and what time intervals will be used.

2. A.N. was sleeping when the fire started and managed to make her way out of the house through thick smoke. You are concerned about possible smoke inhalation. What assessment findings would corroborate this concern?

3. A.N. is very concerned about visible scars. What will you tell her to allay her fears?

4. A.N. is in severe pain. What is the drug of choice for pain relief following burn injury, and how should it be given?

5. A.N.'s burns are to be treated by the open-method with topical application of silver sufadiazine (Silvadene). What is the major drawback to this method of treatment?

6. A special burn diet is ordered for A.N.. She has always gained weight easily and is concerned about the size of the portions. What diet-related teaching will you provide?

7. Tissues under and around A.N.'s burns are severely swollen. She looks at you with tears in her eyes and asks, "Will they stay this way?" What is your answer?

8. Following significant burn injury, the patient is at high risk for infection. What nursing measures will you institute to prevent this?

9. A.N. has one area of circumferential burns on her right lower leg. What complication is she in danger of developing and how will you monitor for it?

Case Study 2

Name: _____ Class/Group: _____ Date: _____

Instructions: All questions apply to this case study. Your response should be brief and to the point. Adequate space has been provided for answers. When asked to provide several answers, they should be listed in order of priority or significance. Do not assume information that is not provided. Please print or write legibly.

You are working evenings on an orthopedic floor. One of your patients, J.O., is a 25-year-old man who was a new admission on day shift. He was involved in a motor vehicle accident (MVA) during a high-speed police chase. His admitting diagnosis is status post (s/p) open reduction and internal fixation of the R femur, which was performed under general anesthesia, multiple rib fractures, sternal bruise, and multiple abrasions. He speaks some English but is more comfortable with his "home" language. He is under arrest for narcotics trafficking, so one wrist is shackled to the bed and he has a guard with him continuously. Another drug dealer has told him "he's coming to get him." Hospital security is aware of the situation.

Your initial assessment reveals stable VS of 116/78, 84, 16, 98.6°F. His only complaint is pain, for which he has a PCA pump. He has crackles in lung bases bilaterally. His abdomen is soft and nontender. He has an indwelling Foley catheter and an nasogastric tube connected to low wall suction. His IV of D_5 LR is infusing in the proximal port of a L subclavian triple lumen catheter, the remaining two ports are heparin locked. His R femur is connected to skeletal traction. The dressing is dry and intact over the incision site.

1. J.O. wants to smoke a cigarette. He usually smokes a pack a day and has had none since the accident. He is irate because the day nurse would not let him smoke. What is your major concern about J.O.'s smoking?

2. J.O.'s right leg is connected to 10 pounds of skeletal traction. As you troubleshoot the system, you note that the ropes are knotted at connection sites, the pulleys have rope running along the center tracts, the leg is slightly flexed at the knee, the leg is 6 inches above the mattress, and the 10-pound weight is resting on the floor. Are any of these findings of concern to you? If so, how would you fix it?

The nurse in the emergency room phones to tell you that J.O.'s immunization status could not be determined when he arrived so no tetanus immunization was given. When you ask J.O. the date of his last tetanus shot, he looks puzzled and asks you what a tetanus shot is. When asking about his childhood, you find that he was born and raised in Colombia. He immigrated to the United States 5 years ago. He does not know if he has ever had a tetanus shot. You inform the physician and he orders diphtheria/tetanus toxoid 0.5 ml IM and Hypertet (tetanus immune globulin) 250 U deep IM.

3.   Why is J.O. getting two injections?

4.   J.O. has a Foley catheter inserted to drain his urine. What should the nurse assess for in relation to the Foley catheter?

5.   While assessing distal to the fractured femur, the nurse notes that his toes are cold to the touch. What other assessment findings should be gathered?

6.   J.O. has an antiembolism stockings ordered for his L leg. What is the rationale for putting stockings on only one leg?

7.   At 1800 J.O.'s guard summons you to his room. J.O. is cold and clammy, groaning, pale, agitated, and slightly confused. VS are 70/palp, 140, 28, 98.0°F. His pulse is weak and thready. His abdomen is painful and appears to be increased in size. You summon the physician. What else can you do?

8.   The physician arrives and wishes to perform a peritoneal lavage. Explain why peritoneal lavage is being done, and describe the procedure.

9.   What are the nursing responsibilities in preparation for this procedure (in order)?

10. The physician begins the diagnostic peritoneal lavage procedure. Upon insertion of the trochar into the abdomen, bright red blood under pressure returns. What happens next?

11. In view of the threat made on J.O.'s life and his vulnerable situation, what precautions should the nursing unit take to protect him?

J.O. recovered for several weeks in the hospital before being sent to jail to await trial. Shortly before his trial date, he was found stabbed to death in his cell. Although there was an investigation, the murder weapon was never found, and no one was ever charged in his death.

Case Study 3

Name: _____ Class/Group: _____ Date: _____

Instructions: All questions apply to this case study. Your response should be brief and to the point. Adequate space has been provided for answers. When asked to provide several answers, they should be listed in order of priority or significance. Do not assume information that is not provided. Please print or write legibly.

You are working on the cardiac unit. One of your patients, J.H., is 52 years old and has had an acute anterior wall myocardial infarction (MI). He is a police detective who is overweight, smokes 2 packs per day, drinks daily, sporadically takes his antihypertensive medication, and is angry that he is in the hospital. He suffered his MI during a heated argument with his wife. He initially blamed her for all of his current problems and refused to cooperate, but he has now consented to participate in the cardiac rehabilitation program. From his barrel chest and history, you also assume he has COPD, although that has not specifically been diagnosed.

Upon arrival at his bedside you note that he is extremely short of breath. He is having difficulty talking and has gurgling respirations and a moist cough. You are surprised to see his IV is empty. He tells you that the nurse told him he could go have a cigarette after his IV antibiotic was finished, so he "opened the valve to make it run faster."

1. You suspect he has pulmonary edema. What other assessment findings would confirm your suspicion?

2. What position will J.H. find most comfortable during this episode?

J.H. has the following medications ordered: furosemide (Lasix) 40 mg IV q6h, potassium (K-Dur) 20 mEq PO bid, digoxin (Lanoxin) 0.25 mg PO qd, lisinopril (Prinovil) 10 mg qd, morphine 2-4 mg IVP prn, 2 L O_2/nc HS and prn. He has not had any medications yet this morning.

3. What medications might you give him before the arrival of the physician? State your rationale.

4. You summon the physician STAT. An additional intravenous dose of Lasix 40 mg is ordered. How fast can Lasix be administered IVP? What is the onset of action?

5. J.H. diureses effectively and begins breathing more comfortably. He does not understand how such a small amount of fluid from his antibiotic could cause such big problems. He asks you to explain it.

6. In view of his recent diuresis, what 2 lab values would you especially need to monitor?

7. Once J.H. has recovered from his episode of pulmonary edema, you decide to take advantage of the "teachable moment" to reinforce the concept of fluid overload. List 3 other ways J.H. can cause an overload of fluid in his body.

8. J.H. tells you that his favorite things to eat and drink are ham sandwiches, peanuts, coffee, beer, iced tea, apple juice, colas, and milk. Which ones can he continue to eat or drink on a low-sodium cardiac prevention diet?

9. J.H. becomes short of breath while he is walking with you. He panics and is absolutely certain he is going into pulmonary edema again. You believe he is suffering from dyspnea on exertion. Explain the difference between dyspnea on exertion and pulmonary edema.

10. Pulmonary function tests are performed while J.H. is in the hospital, and COPD is confirmed. From J.H.'s history, what factor probably contributed to both his cardiac and pulmonary disease?

J.H.'s wife has had enough. She goes home, throws out all the ashtrays, and comes into his room announcing he will either quit smoking or she is going to throw him out. J.H. tries to get sympathy from you. "Sorry, Marlboro Man," you tell him, "She's right this time, and you're on your own." He glares at you both for a few minutes, then shrugs and pulls out his "secret stash" of cigarettes and his lighter, hands them to you, and tells you it's OK to trash them. "Guess what?" you cheerfully inform him, "We've got a smoking cessation class starting this afternoon and it's going to be full of a bunch of tough guys like you!"

Case Study 4

Name: _____ Class/Group: _____ Date: _____

Instructions: All questions apply to this case study. Your response should be brief and to the point. Adequate space has been provided for answers. When asked to provide several answers, they should be listed in order of priority or significance. Do not assume information that is not provided. Please print or write legibly.

You are working on a telemetry unit and have just received a transfer from the intensive care unit. The 50-year-old male patient, T.A., had a repair of an abdominal aortic aneurysm (AAA) measuring 8 cm in diameter. This is his second day postop. He is an attorney with a very active practice. He considered himself to be healthy before diagnosis of the aneurysm, although he took medication for gastric hyperacidity. He has had progressive weakness of his lower extremities and decreasing urine output since surgery. T.A. also has a 10-year history of type II diabetes mellitus; he has been requiring animal-based insulin the last 6 months to keep his glucose levels under control.

1. T.A. is very concerned about the leg weakness since his surgery. He states, "If I had knowm this was going to happen, I never would have agreed to the surgery. I was fine before. I'd still be fine now if I hadn't been operated on, wouldn't I?" Your response based on the knowledge of aortic aneurysm should be:

2. You are performing your initial assessment of T.A.'s legs. What findings should you record?

3. Four hours after admission to your floor you note that T.A. has had a urine output of 75 ml of dark amber urine. You examine the catheter and tubing for obstructions and there are none. What other assessment data should you gather to determine if a problem exists?

4. Laboratory tests reveal renal damage. T.A. is placed on a fluid restriction and a renal diet. T.A. asks what he is going to be able to eat on his diet. You reply:

5. T.A. has a dialysis catheter inserted into his left subclavian vein. You are preparing to administer an intravenous antibiotic and find that his only other intravenous access, a peripheral line, is obstructed. What should you do?

6. Upon return from his first dialysis, T.A. complains of headache and nausea, is slightly confused, restless, and has an elevated blood pressure. You suspect disequilibrium phenomenon. You notify the physician. What nursing measures can you institute at this point?

7. T.A. has an episode of severe vomiting. His abdominal wound dehisces, and a loop of his intestines eviscerates. Another staff member has summoned the doctor. What care should you render before the physician's arrival?

8. You are concerned that the weakness in Mr. Andrew's legs may result in muscle atrophy. What nursing interventions can you take to prevent this?

A sliding scale human recombinant insulin plan has been instituted, but T.A.'s glucose levels have been ranging from 62 to 387 mg/dl. "That's funny," he tells, you. "You're giving about the same amount about the same times as I gave it to myself at home. I don't understand why it's not working!" You explain to him that the dialysis and the surgery both profoundly affect his insulin needs. In addition, although it may look similar in the syringe, he is getting a different dose of insulin than he has been getting at home.

9. Based on recent findings contrasting the metabolism of human insulin versus animal insulin sources, explain why T.A. may be having trouble regulating his glucose levels.

10. T.A.'s wound is not healing. You call the enterostomal therapy (ET) RN to evaluate what can be done. After looking at T.A.'s wound, he looks at T.A.'s chart, sighs, and points to the glucose levels. "Here's your problem," he says. "The way this is going, he'll never heal." Based on recent findings in diabetes management, explain what he means. What other health care professionals may help you with T.A.'s glucose regulation?

Case Study 5

Name: _____ *Class/Group:* _____ *Date:* _____

Instructions: All questions apply to this case study. Your response should be brief and to the point. Adequate space has been provided for answers. When asked to provide several answers, they should be listed in order of priority or significance. Do not assume information that is not provided. Please print or write legibly.

T.M., a long-haul trucker, has arrived as an emergency department admission. He has a history of chronic bronchitis that has been controlled on an outpatient basis for the last 10 years. After a 10-day road trip, he noted that his left leg was swollen and painful. A scan revealed a deep vein thrombosis (DVT) of the left leg (a 24-cm clot in the left femoral vein). His admission VS are 190/110, 76, 24, 100°F. His admission assessment shows barrel chest; male pattern obesity ("beer belly"); heart sounds that are distant secondary to lung sounds; rhonchi and wheezes intermittently in all lung fields; enlarged palpable liver; and a left lower leg that is red, edematous, warm, and significantly larger than the right. He has been told by his physician to quit smoking, drinking, lose weight, and increase exercise. He has decreased his drinking to weekends when he is not on the road and has switched to light beer. But, he still smokes 2 packs per day and remains overweight. He takes theophylline (Theodur) 300 mg PO q8h and uses an ipratropium (Atrovent) inhaler q4h prn to help keephis COPD under control.

1. Upon admission, T.M. states, "I just don't know how this happened....I've been taking my drugs and cut back on my beer. I've even lost 10 pounds. This healthy living stuff is overrated!" List and explain his risk factors for DVT versus the primary contributing factor to his DVT.

2. T.M. wants to know why his liver is enlarged when he has just about quit drinking. How are you going to explain this to him?

3. The physician ordered total bed rest. T.M. says he can't possibly stay in bed all the time, he has to go outside to smoke and he absolutely has to go to the bathroom. He tries to bargain with you not to get up to smoke if he can go to the bathroom. He thinks you are being unreasonable and asks why you won't at least let him get up to the bathroom. How are you going to respond?

4. T.M. is placed on 2 L O_2/nc, a heparin drip, an IV antibiotic, and his usual COPD medications. Four days after admission, his wife calls you to the room "because he's acting weird." When you arrive, you observe he is very confused; he was lucid an hour ago. What should you do?

You note decreased strength and movement in the L side of his body. He also has a mild facial droop on the L side of his face. The physician arrives and orders a STAT CT scan of the head with and without contrast.

5. According to his wife, T.M. has no drug allergies; he's only allergic to shrimp. What significance does this allergy have?

6. An x-ray transporter arrives to take T.M. to x-ray. Additional floor personnel who could go to the x-ray include 3 certified nurses aides (CNAs), licensed practical nurse (LPN), 3 RNs, and the physician. Who should accompany T.M. to x-ray and why?

7. CT scan reveals a right hemispheric cerebral thrombosis from an embolus. On return from the CT scan you observe his level of consciousness has decreased, and he no longer responds to questions. Although the doctor explained the findings to her, his wife keeps asking you when he is going to wake up. What should you do?

8. If he survives this current crisis, which complication of CVA is T.M. at greatest risk of acquiring?

Case Study 6

You are working nights on an inpatient geriatric unit. An 82-year-old woman, M.B., is admitted from an extended care facility with urosepsis, Alzheimer's disease, and a history of hypertension and CVA. Her right side is flaccid. She does not communicate, moans when in pain, and hits, kicks, and claws with her left arm and leg when disturbed. Her initial assessment shows emaciation and multiple pressure ulcers. She has an indwelling Foley catheter and one peripheral IV of D_5 NS at 75 ml/h. Her initial VS are 86/50, 108, 24, 104.6°F. Her initial WBC is 34.2 mm³.

1. Four hours after admission you note that M.B.'s Foley catheter has not drained any urine. You cannot begin her antibiotics until you collect a urine culture. What should you do?

2. M.B. has 2 intravenous antibiotics, gentamicin (Garamycin) and ticarcillin (Ticar), ordered for 1000. Her morning serum creatinine is 3.2 mg/dl. Her admission serum creatinine was 2.0. Which medication can you safely give?

3. M.B.'s diet is "mechanical soft." The certified nursing assistant (CNA) tells you that M.B. often spits food during feeding. She also becomes agitated and tries to hit and kick the CNA during meals. Her total intake is less than 25% of the food she is supposed to receive. You believe she may be suffering from protein caloric malnutrition. What assessment findings would you gather to support this?

4. M.B. has a PEG tube inserted and is started on continuous tube feedings at 100 ml/h. During your morning assessment you note that her gastric residual is 175 ml. There are no specific orders regarding residual amount. What should you do?

5. M.B. is at high risk for pulmonary aspiration of her tube feedings. What nursing measures can decrease the chances for this complication?

6. M.B. has a large, stage IV decubitus ulcer over her sacrum and stage II decubitus ulcers over both trochanters. You are initiating a turning schedule for M.B.. What would be the most effective positions and schedule?

7. The enterostomal therapy nurse orders Elase ointment to the sacral decubitus followed by wet-to-moist dressing. What observations are important to note following dressing changes?

8. What could you do to improve M.B's quality of life?

One of the CNAs at the extended care facility said M.B. always "perked up" when their therapy dog, Cindy, came for a visit. Although hospital policy prohibited dogs (except for companion and helper dogs) visiting in patients' rooms, special permission was obtained for Cindy to visit M.B. "It was miraculous," the afternoon nurse told her colleague at report, "M.B. perked up and smiled for the first time since she came here. She petted that dog for the longest time and seemed more relaxed and cooperative afterward than you ever could imagine. Maybe all she needed was a little loving. Anyway, they left a picture of Cindy for her to keep on her bedside stand. It seems to have a calming effect on her."

Case Study 7

You are admitting a 30-year-old woman, J.L., to your telemetry unit with the diagnosis of status postcardiac transplantation and fever of unknown origin (FUO). She was healthy until the birth of her only child at age 27. She developed idiopathic cardiomyopathy following childbirth and underwent cardiac transplantation at age 29. There is a family history of early death from "heart problems."

1. Admitting has assigned J.L. to a semiprivate room. Her roommate is on day 4 of intravenous antibiotic treatment for pneumonia and now has a near normal WBC level. Is this assignment appropriate? What is your response?

2. Fever is a sign of 2 major complications of organ transplantation. What are they?

3. What other signs and symptoms of organ rejection should the nurse assess for in this patient?

4. What other signs and symptoms of sepsis should the nurse assess for in J.L.?

5. While you are assessing J.L., she tells you that she always urinates frequently, because of her diuretics. However, she has experienced burning with urination for the last 2 days. You wish to collect a urine specimen for laboratory analysis. What do you suspect may be causing the burning, and what type of urine specimen should you obtain?

6. The physician tells you that J.L. is to be started on antibiotics as quickly as possible. She has just had a PICC line inserted, and her first dose of intravenous antibiotics has just arrived from the pharmacy. Is there other information that you would like to know before you begin her antibiotics?

7. J.L. says she has complained to her physician that she is constantly short of breath running after her 3-year-old. She says her physician told her that this is to be expected but did not tell her why. Why does she become dyspneic with exertion?

8. J.L. tells you that her husband's parents have given her child their cat because they play so well together. She jokingly says, "They gave him the play and me the work! My husband is going to have to help. I'm not up to looking after a cat, too." What job does her husband need to do?

9. You would like to teach J.L. some practical things she can do to protect herself from infection. List 5. (*Hint:* this would include many of the same things cancer patients on chemotherapy are taught.)

CHAPTER 11. EMERGENCY SITUATIONS

Case Study 1

The American Heart Association has two different classifications of certifications, one for lay people and one for all health care providers. As a nursing student you should use the health care provider guidelines to answer the following questions.

You are on duty in an extended care facility, when you enter a patient's room and find the patient unconscious and not breathing. The patient's meal tray is in front of her, and you notice part of an orange on it.

1. What is the first action you should take?

The patient does not respond.

2. What would you do next?

3. How would you open the airway?

The patient is not breathing.

4. What is your next action?

After attempting rescue breathing, the patient's chest does not rise.

5. What should you do next?

You detect no obstruction.

6. What should you do next?

After repeated maneuvers, the situation remains unchanged.

7. What should your next action be?

The paramedics arrive and attempt to manually ventilate the patient with a bag-valve mask device. They are unable to ventilate the patient's lungs. They then attempt to intubate the patient. While visualizing with the laryngoscope, the paramedic notices dentures and a piece of orange in the patient's airway.

8. How could this obstruction have occurred?

The obstructions were removed, the patient was intubated, manually ventilated, and transported to the hospital. She suffered a cardiac arrest in the ambulance and all attempts to resuscitate were unsuccessful. The patient was pronounced dead on arrival at the hospital.

9. What 3 could have been taken in the above scenario that may have averted this outcome. List preventive measures first.

Case Study 2

You are the nurse on a medical unit taking care of a 40-year-old man, T.Z., who has been admitted with peptic ulcer disease (PUD) secondary to chronic alcoholism. You enter T.Z.'s room and find him having a grand mal (tonic-clonic) seizure.

1. List 5 things you would do.

   Note: Placing any objects, including an airway into the patient's mouth at this point is contraindicated, due to the possibility of patient or caregiver harm.

T.Z.'s seizure activity does not appear to be subsiding and he is becoming cyanotic. The physician is notified and orders diazepam (Valium) 5 to 10 mg IV until seizure activity subsides.

2. What is the rationale for giving T.Z. diazepam?

3. What is status epilepticus?

4. What would you be particularly alert for when giving diazepam intravenously (list 3)?

By the time the physician arrives, T.Z.'s seizure activity has not subsided. The physician administers an additional 10 mg of diazepam, without effect. Fifteen minutes has elapsed since you found T.Z. having seizure activity.

5. What is the significance of this?

The physician decides to administer vecuronium (Norcuron) and intubate T.Z.

6.   What is vecuronium and why is it being administered to T.Z.?

T.Z. has been intubated; the physician orders 600 mg phenobarbital IV and transport to ICU.

7.   What is the rationale behind giving phenobarbital?

8.   List 2 nursing diagnoses for T.Z.

9.   Given T.Z.'s above history, state at least 2 possible causes for his grand mal seizure.

T.Z's seizure was successfully treated with diazepam and phenobarbital, and he has had no further seizure activity. As you are writing up his release papers, you overhear T.Z. telling his girlfriend to have his car brought to the hospital so he can drive home.

10. How should you respond to this situation?

Case Study 3

It is 0800, and the outpatient clinic where you work as an RN has just opened. R.W., a 40-year-old man, hops into the clinic complaining of severe pain and swelling in his right lower leg. He tells you he was walking between two cars the night before, when one of the cars was backed up, catching his lower leg between the bumpers. He states he didn't think it was "hurt that bad" and went home to wash the abrasions. He woke up at approximately 0400, and states "My leg was killing me."

1. How would you transport R.W. to the examining room?

R.W. is placed in the examining room and asked to remove his trousers and put on a gown. R.W. is unable to lay his leg on the exam table without pain. You observe that his right lower leg is grossly edematous and pale.

2. What should your next priority be?

There are no pulses in the distal extremity, sensation is diminished, the extremity is cold to touch, and any movement is extremely painful.

3. What should your next action be?

The physician is with another patient, and asks you to wait a minute.

4. How should you respond?

After assessing the patient, the physician determines that R.W. should be transported to the nearest ED. The clinic physician notifies the ED physician that R.W. is coming in by ambulance with possible compartment syndrome of the right lower leg.

5. Explain the pathophysiology of compartment syndrome and clarify its significance.

6. How is compartment syndrome treated?

7. While waiting for the ambulance, R.W. starts to tell you "one-leg" jokes. How will you respond?

8. How would you manage the fasciotomy once it has been performed?

Given that this is a crush injury, the physician orders a urine for myoglobin on R.W.

9. What is the rationale behind this order?

10. How is rhabdomyolysis treated?

After an uneventful 5-day stay on the surgical unit, R.W. is being discharged to home care services and has been referred for physical therapy.

11. As you question him about his living conditions, you discover that R.W. lives alone in a third story apartment; there are no elevators. What other information do you need from him in preparation for discharge?

Case Study 4

T.R. is a 22-year-old college senior who lives in the dormitory. His friend finds him wandering aimlessly about the campus appearing pale and sweaty. He engages T.R. in conversation and walks him to the campus medical clinic where you are on duty. It is 1050. He explains to you how he found T.R., and states that he knows T.R. is a diabetic and takes insulin. T.R. is not wearing a medical warning tag.

1. What do you think is going on with T.R.?

2. List 2 nursing diagnoses for T.R.

3. What is the first action you would take?

4. Because the glucometer reading is 50 mg/dl, what would your next action be?

5. When you enter the room to administer the orange juice, T.R. is unresponsive. What should your next action be?

6. T.R. is breathing at 16 breaths per minute, has a pulse of 85 and regular, but remains unresponsive. What should your next action be if (1) your clinic is well-equipped for emergencies, and (2) your clinic has no emergency supplies? *Since this is an outpatient setting, your resources may vary:*

7. What questions would you ask to find out what precipitated these events?

T.R. tells you he took 35 units human NPH and 12 units of regular human insulin at 0745. He says he was late to class so he just grabbed an apple on the way. He adds this has happened twice in the past, but he recognized it and treated it with candy and then ate a meal. He says he is on a 2000 calorie ADA diet (newer research is calling into question the older "ADA calorie diet" approach, but it still is commonly taught and used).

8. Based on your knowledge of different types of insulin, when would you expect T.R. to experience an insulin reaction?

9. In discussing your teaching plan with T.R., list at least 4 important points that you would stress.

Case Study 5

You are on duty in the ED when a "Code Blue" is called overhead. As the code nurse, you grab the crash cart and run to the code, which is in the employee lounge of the operating room. On the couch you find a nurse unconscious, cyanotic, and barely breathing. Her scrub shirt has been cut off, and you attach ECG leads to her chest. Her pulse is 45; respirations are 8 and shallow. She is intubated, an intravenous line is started with 0.9% NaCl, and she is given an ampule of 50 ml D_5W, 0.4 mg naloxone (Narcan), and 0.5 mg atropine IVP. Her respirations improve slightly, and pulse increases to 56. She is transported to the ED.

1.   What is the purpose of giving the 3 above-mentioned drugs in this case?

After additional naloxone, the patient woke up and was extubated.

2.   What additional information do you want to know?

In response to your questions, Z.H. tells you that she had taken fentanyl IM. She then asks you to call a friend to come stay with her.

3.   What information would you give her friend over the phone?

4.   The friend asks you what is wrong. How do you respond?

5.   Identify 5 nursing diagnoses that may apply in this situation.

Z.H. is admitted to the ICU for 24-hour observation and then transferred to the chemical dependency unit.

6.   What is chemical dependency?

One of Z.H.'s colleagues calls on the phone to ask how she is. She tells you that she thought something was wrong with Z.H. because her behavior was so erratic, but "I had no idea it was drugs. I didn't think Z.H. would ever do anything like that!" Keep in mind that patient confidentiality extends to health care professionals not directly involved in Z.H.'s care. You cannot give information on how Z.H. is doing.

7.   What is the profile of an impaired nurse (list 5 characteristics).

8.   What 4 are problems associated with impaired nurses who are practicing?

Z.H. asks her nurse what is going to happen to her career.

9.   What are the regulatory issues r/t impaired nurses that will guide your response (list at least 5)?

Z.H. successfully completed treatment and continues to practice as a nurse. She is now serving as a sponsor for another nurse undergoing treatment for chemical dependency.

Case Study 6

J.R. is a 28-year-old man who is doing home repairs. He falls from the top of a 6 foot step ladder, striking his head on a large rock. He experiences momentary loss of consciousness. By the time his neighbor gets to him, he is conscious but bleeding profusely from a laceration over the R temporal area. The neighbor drives him to the ED of your hospital. As the nurse, you immediately apply a cervical collar, lay him on a stretcher, and take J.R. to a treatment room.

1. What steps should you take to assess J.R.?

2. List at least 5 components of a neuro exam.

You complete your neuro exam and find the following: GCS 15, PERRLA, and has full sensation. He complains of a headache; he is becoming increasingly lethargic.

3. As the radiology technician performs a portable cross table lateral c-spine x-ray, J.R. begins to speak incoherently and appears to drift off to sleep. What is the next action you would take?

You find J.R. has become unresponsive to verbal stimuli and responds to painful stimuli by abnormally flexing his extremities (decorticate movement). He has no verbal response. The right pupil is larger than the left, and does not respond to light.

4. What is J.R.'s Glasgow coma scale (GCS) score at this time? Indicate what this means.

5. Based on his GSC score, what are the next steps you should take?

6.   What is the significance of the dilated and fixed pupil on the right?

The physician orders 500 ml of 25% mannitol solution IV.

7.   What is mannitol, and why is it being used on J.R.?

J.R. is transported to CT scan where he is found to have a large epidural hematoma on the right with a hemispheric shift to the left. He will be taken to the OR from CT scan for evacuation of a right epidural hematoma.

While en route from the CT scan to the OR, the physician instructs the respiratory therapist to initiate hyperventilation of the patient to "blow off more CO_2."

8.   What is the rationale for this action?

9.   Explain at least 6 nursing interventions you would use to prevent increased ICP in the first 48 postoperative hours.

While he is in surgery, J.R.'s family arrives at the ED. They ask that their faith healer anoint J.R. and pray over him.

10.   What should the nurse say?

Case Study 7

B.J. is a 34-year-old woman who has been thrown from a galloping horse in a remote area. She was flown to the trauma center by helicopter from a rural hospital with spinal cord compression due to spinal fracture and disk fragments in her lumbar spine. Her cervical spine is free from injury. She arrives strapped to a rigid backboard and begins to vomit.

1. What would you do to keep B.J. from aspirating?

2. What would you do to assess B.J.?

You find that B.J. is hypotensive and bradycardic. She has an IV of 1000 ml LR with a large-bore catheter at 75 ml/h.

3. What is causing the hypotension and bradycardia?

The neurosurgeon arrives in the ED and examines B.J. He finds her areflexic below the lumbar region of the spinal cord. There is absence of sweating in the region, and no sensation below the level of the lesion. He writes the following orders: CT scan of the spine; myelogram; prepare for surgery; admit to ICU; 10 mg dexamethasone (Decadron) IV now.

4. Why did the physician order both a CT scan and a myelogram? Differentiate between the diagnostic value of each.

5. What is dexamethasone, and why is it being used on B.J.?

6. List 5 nursing diagnoses for B.J.

7. What are complications and problems associated with spinal cord shock (minimum of 7)?

8. How would you detect complications from spinal cord shock (list 6)?

9. What are 8 interventions that could be initiated to prevent or treat complications from spinal cord shock?

B.J. went to surgery directly from x-ray for decompression of her spinal cord, and was admitted to ICU on absolute bed rest. From ICU she was transferred to the surgical unit, fitted for a back brace, and began physiotherapy. After undergoing surgery for a bone graft and spinal fusion, she was transferred to a rehabilitation facility. After months of intense physiotherapy, B.J. regained the use of her legs and basic functioning and was discharged to home.

Case Study 8

You are working on the intermediate cardiac care unit in a large hospital. You are taking care of R.J. who was admitted for a chest contusion he sustained in an auto accident and fractured 4th and 5th ribs on the left side. About 2000, his wife runs up to you at the nurse's station and says "I think my husband just had a heart attack. Come quick!" She follows you into his room, where you find him face down on the floor. He is breathing, is cyanotic from the neck up, and his pulse is very weak.

1.   What should your first action be?

2.   Suddenly, you remember R.J.'s wife, who is anxiously hovering over you in the room. What are you going to do?

The code team arrives. R.J.'s trauma surgeon is making rounds on your unit when the code is called, and he runs to the room. R.J. is intubated, and the NS lock is changed to an IV of LR. The trauma surgeon recognizes Beck's triad and calls for a cardiac needle and syringe. He inserts the needle below the xiphoid process and aspirates 50 ml of unclotted blood.

3.   What is Beck's triad and what causes it?

4.   Explain the rationale for the surgeon performing a pericardiocentesis.

R.J. is transferred to the thoracic intensive care unit for observation.

5.   List 3 nursing diagnoses for R.J.

6.   As the team prepares R.J.'s transfer, you go to find R.J.'s wife to tell her what has happened. Briefly, and in everyday terms, how would you explain what happend to her husband?

7.   As you both get up to leave, Mrs. J. suddenly turns pale and says she feels very dizzy. What are you going to do?

Case Study 9

You are working in the ED when a patient comes in having an allergic reaction to bee pollen she has eaten. She brought the jar of bee pollen with her. Your nurse colleague, curious as to how bee pollen tastes, ingests a small amount. A few minutes later your colleague begins to experience itching in her throat and ears, hives, and mild respiratory distress. The respiratory distress rapidly progresses to audible wheezing. You notice that your colleague appears to be in distress.

1. What do you think is wrong with your colleague?

2. Given that your colleague is having a possible allergic reaction, what actions should you take (list 6)?

3. What is the rationale behind giving the medications you identified in answer 2 above? Indicate their usual dosages.

4. Identify 3 nursing diagnoses for B.J.

The nurse begins to improve. She states that the itching has subsided and the hives are fading. She reports that she no longer has acute shortness of breath. On auscultation of her lungs, you note that the wheezing has resolved. She wants to return to work.

5. Is it appropriate to allow her to return to duty? Why?

A decision is made to discharge the nurse to her home.

6. What issues should you address in discharge teaching of this nurse (list 3)?

7. Should you allow the nurse to drive herself home? Why?

A friend was called to come and drive your colleague home, and she was discharged. She lived to nurse another day.

Case Study 10

You are working in an outpatient clinic when a mother brings in her 20-year-old-daughter, C.J., who has type I diabetes mellitus and has just returned from a trip to Mexico. She's had a 3-day FUO (fever of undetermined origin), and diarrhea with N&V. She has been unable to eat and has tolerated only sips of fluid. Because she has been unable to eat, she has not taken her insulin.

Because C.J. is unsteady, you bring her to the examining room in a wheelchair. While assisting her onto the examining table, you note that her skin is very warm and flushed. Her respirations are deep and rapid, and her breath is foul smelling. C.J. is drowsy and unable to answer your questions. Her mother states "she keeps telling me she's so thirsty, but she can't keep anything down."

1.   What additional information do you need to elicit from C.J.'s mother (list 4)?

2.   Describe the pathophysiology of diabetic ketoacidosis.

3.   Explain the patient's presenting signs and symptoms (list 6).

4. Her current VS are 90/50, 124, 36 and deep; temperature is 101.3° F (tympanic temp). Are these vital signs appropriate for a woman of C.J.'s age? Why or why not? Discuss your rationale.

5. Write 3 nursing diagnoses for C.J.

A decision has been made to transport C.J. by ambulance to the local ED. After evaluating C.J., the ED physician writes the following orders.

6. Carefully review each order to determine if it is appropriate or inappropriate as written. Place an "A" in the space provided if appropriate; place an "I" in the space provided if inappropriate and <u>underline</u> the inappropriate part. Explain why it is inappropriate and correct the order.

    ___ 1000 ml LR IV STAT.
    ___ Give 36 units lente and 20 units regular insulin SC (sub-Q) now.
    ___ CBC with differential; Chem 20 (electrolytes, glucose, enzymes); blood cultures x 2 sites; clean catch urine for UA and C&S; stool for ova and parasites, *C. difficile* toxin, and C&S; serum lactate, ketone, and osmolality; ABGs on room air.
    ___ 1800 calorie ADA diet.
    ___ Ambulate qid.
    ___ Tylenol 650 mg (10 gr) PO.
    ___ Lasix 60 mg IVP now.
    ___ Urine output every hour.
    ___ VS q shift.

All orders have been corrected and initiated. C.J. has received fluid resuscitation and is on a sliding scale insulin drip via infusion pump. Her latest glucose was 347 mg/dl.

   7.   What is the rationale behind using an infusion pump for the insulin drip?

C.J. is ready for transport to the medical ICU. C.J.'s mother is beginning to realize that C.J. is more acutely ill than she thought. She leaves the room and begins to cry.

   8.   How would you handle this situation?

   9.   C.J.'s mother asks where she can get more information on how C.J. can control her diabetes. What are some resources she may find useful?

C.J. was transported to the MICU in slightly improved condition. She continued to improve, and was discharged from the hospital 3 days later.

Case Study 11

Name: _____ Class/Group: _____ Date: _____

Instructions: All questions apply to this case study. Your response should be brief and to the point. Adequate space has been provided for answers. When asked to provide several answers, they should be listed in order of priority or significance. Do not assume information that is not provided. Please print or write legibly.

You are the nurse on duty on the intermediate care unit and you are scheduled to take the next admission. The ED nurse calls to give you the following report, "This is Barb in the ED and we have a 42-year-old man with lower GI bleeding. He is a sandblaster with a 12-year history of silicosis. He is taking 40 mg of prednisone per day. During the night, he developed severe diarrhea. He was unable to get out of bed fast enough and had a large maroon-colored stool (hematochezia) in the bed. His wife 'freaked' and called the paramedics. He has been seen here and is coming to you. His VS are stable: 110/64, 110, 28, and he's a little agitated. His temperature is 36.8° C. He hasn't had any stools since admission but his rectal exam was guaiac positive and he is pale but not diaphoretic. We have him on 5 L O_2/nc. We started a 16-gauge IV with LR at 125/hour. He has an 18-gauge Salem sump to continuous low suction; the drainage is guaiac negative. We have done a CBC with differential, Chem 20, PT/PTT, and a T&C for 4 units PRCs and a UA. He's all ready for you."

1.   How should you prepare for this patient's arrival?

K.L. arrives on your unit. As you help him transfer from the ED stretcher to the bed, K.L. becomes very dyspneic and expels 800 ml of maroon stool.

2.   What are the first 3 actions you should take?

K.L. reports that he is getting nauseated, but not thirsty. VS are 106/68, 116, 32.

3.   What additional interventions would you need to institute?

The ABG results are as follows (these results reflect values at sea level): pH 7.45; $PaCO_2$ 33 mm Hg; PaO_2 65 mm Hg; HCO_3 23 mEq/L; BE +1.0 mEq/L; SaO_2 91%.

4.   Interpret the preceding ABGs. What do they tell you?

The gastroenterologist was notified by K.L.'s physician and arrives on the unit to perform a colonoscopy and endoscopy. You are going to be giving K.L. midazolam (Versed) and meperidine (Demerol) IV during the procedures.

5. Given the above history, what do you think significantly contributed to the GI bleed?

6. What are midazolam and meperidine, and why are they being given to K.L.?

During the colonoscopy, K.L. begins passing large amounts of bright red blood. He becomes more pale and diaphoretic, and begins to have an altered level of consciousness.

7. Identify 5 immediate interventions you should initiate.

8. List 4 nursing diagnoses for K.L.

K.L. has been stabilized with fluids, blood, and FFP. There has been no further evidence of active bleeding. He received ranitidine (Zantac) 50 mg IV push, and is receiving an infusion of 8 mg/h via infusion pump.

9. Later, when he seems to be feeling better, K.L. tells you he's really embarrassed about the mess he made for you. How are you going to respond to him?

It was concluded that the GI hemorrhage was prednisone-induced. The physician will discharge K.L. and attempt to decrease his maintenance dose of prednisone while monitoring his respiratory status (the prednisone is being used to suppress the progression of silicosis).

Case Study 12

S.K., a 51-year-old roofer, was admitted to the hospital 3 days ago after falling 15 feet from a roof. He sustained bilateral fractured wrists, and an open fracture of the left tibia/fibula. He was taken to surgery for open reduction and internal fixation (ORIF) of all his fractures. He is recovering on your orthopedic unit. You have instructions to begin getting him out of bed and into the chair today. When you enter the room to get S.K. into the chair, you noticed that he is very agitated and dyspneic, and says to you, "My chest hurts real bad. I can't breathe."

1.   Identify 5 possible reasons for S.K.'s symptoms.

You auscultate S.K.'s breath sounds. You find that they are diminished in the LLL. S.K. is diaphoretic, tachypneic, and has circumoral cyanosis. His apical pulse is irregular and 110 beats per minute.

2.   List in order of priority 3 actions you should take next.

The physician orders the following: arterial blood gases (ABGs), chest x-ray (CXR), ECG, and ventilation/perfusion (V/Q) lung scan. The blood gas results come back as follows (these results reflect values at sea level): pH 7.47, $PaCO_2$ 33.6 mm Hg, PaO_2 52 mm Hg, HCO_3 24.2 mEq/L, BE -3.4 mEq/L, SaO_2 83%, and A-a gradient 32 mm Hg.

3.   What is your interpretation of the blood gases? Give your rationale.

4.   Based on the ABGs and your assessment findings, what do you think is wrong with S.K.?

5. List 3 nursing diagnoses for S.K.

The physician writes the following orders for S.K.:

___ Transfer to MICU.

___ Heparin 20,000 units IVP now, and 20,000 units in 1000 ml/D_5W to run at 1000 units per hour.

___ PT and PTT every 4 hours. Call house officer with results.

___ 3 L O_2/nc

___ PCA pump with morphine sulfate: loading dose 10 mg; dose 2 mg.; lockout time 15 minutes; maximum 4-hour dose 30 mg.

___ Streptokinase, 250,000 IU IV over 30 minutes, then 100,000 IU per hour x 48 hours.

___ Solucortef 1 g IV now.

___ Albuterol (Proventil) MDI (metered-dose inhaler), 2 puffs q6h.

6. Of the orders *listed above*, identify inappropriate orders by placing a check mark (✓) in the space provided. Give a rationale for your decision.

All orders have been corrected. S.K.'s V/Q scan indicated a pulmonary embolism in the LLL, and antithrombolytic therapy was initiated. Repeat ABGs show the following values (these results reflect values at sea level): pH 7.45, $PaCO_2$ 35 mm Hg, PaO_2 82 mm Hg, HCO_3 24 mEq/L, BE -2.4 mEq/L, SaO_2 90%, A-a gradient 28 mm Hg.

7. What do these gases generally indicate?

The physician orders Lasix 20 mg IV now.

8. Why do you think the physician ordered furosemide (Lasix) for S.K.?

S.K. was watched very closely for the next several days for the onset of pulmonary edema. Thrombolytic therapy, oxygen, pulse oximetry, daily chest x-rays and blood gas analysis, and pain management were continued. When he was stable, S.K. was transferred back to your orthopedic unit.

9. The next day, S.K. suddenly exploded and threw the physical therapist out of his room. He yelled, "I'm sick and tired of having everyone tell me what to do." How are you going to deal with this situation?

Case Study 13

Name: _____ Class/Group: _____ Date: _____

Instructions: All questions apply to this case study. Your response should be brief and to the point. Adequate space has been provided for answers. When asked to provide several answers, they should be listed in order of priority or significance. Do not assume information that is not provided. Please print or write legibly.

D., a 38-year-old woman diagnosed with ruptured appendix, was hospitalized for an appendectomy. She developed peritonitis and was discharged 9 days later with a left peripherally-inserted central catheter (PICC line) to home care for IV antibiotic therapy. You work for the home care department for the hospital. You have been assigned to D.'s case, and this is your first home visit to her. You are to do a full assessment on D. During the assessment, you notice a large ecchymotic area over the right upper arm. You question her about the bruise and she tells you, "the nurses took my blood pressure so many times it bruised."

1.   Do you accept D.'s explanation? Why or why not?

In examining D. further, you find a fine, nonraised, dark red rash over her trunk.

2.   What questions would you ask D. to elicit additional information?

D. hadn't noticed the rash before you pointed it out. The rash does not itch or cause pain. She has never had one like it before.

3.   What other information would you want to gather?

The wound is not discolored or draining; the abdomen is not tender to deep palpation. There is oozing of serosanguinous fluid around the PICC insertion site. The rash is confined to the trunk. You have made a decision to call the physician regarding your assessment findings.

4.   What vital information would you relay to the physician?

The physician orders blood to be drawn for coagulation studies and a CBC with differential. He says he would like to evaluate D. for disseminated intravascular coagulation (DIC).

5.   What laboratory tests would you expect to see performed in coagulation studies?

You give D. her antibiotic, draw her blood, and take it to the lab. You return 6 hours later to administer another dose of antibiotics. D. greets you at the door very upset and ushers you to the bathroom where you find blood in the toilet. She tells you that she has been urinating blood for the past 2 or 3 hours. She also shows you a tissue in which she has bloody-appearing sputum. She tells you she has been coughing up blood. You notify the physician who instructs you call 911 and get the patient to the ED immediately. You call the ED and give report to the triage nurse on duty.

6.   What are you going to tell the triage nurse?

7.   Are the patient's presenting signs and symptoms consistent with DIC? Explain.

The following labs were prolonged: PT, PTT, split fibrin products, and D dimer. The following labs were decreased: platelets, platelet aggregation time, clot retraction time, and fibrinogen level. CBC is all within normal range, with the exception of the WBC, which is 12.5 mm^3, and platelet count, which is 46 mm^3. D. is diagnosed with DIC.

8.   List 4 nursing diagnoses associated with DIC.

9. List at least 3 priority needs for D.

D. was stabilized with oxygen, fluids, and blood products, and medication therapy was initiated. She was transferred to the ICU in guarded condition.

Case Study 14

You are the trauma nurse working in a busy tertiary care facility. You receive a call from the paramedics that they are en route to your facility with the victim of multiple gunshot wounds to the chest and abdomen. The paramedics have started two large-bore IV lines with LR, O_2 by mask at 15 L/minute. The patient has a sucking chest wound on the left and a wound in the upper right quadrant of the abdomen. Vital signs are 80/36, 140, 42. The patient is diaphoretic, very pale, and confused. ETA (estimated time of arrival) is 4 minutes.

1. List at least 6 things you are going to do to prepare for this patient's arrival.

On arrival to the ED, your patient, B.W., is cyanotic and in severe respiratory distress. When he is transferred to the trauma stretcher, you notice that there is an occlusive dressing over the sucking chest wound. It is taped down on all sides.

2. Is taping the occlusive dressing on all sides appropriate? Explain.

3. Who usually responds to a trauma code and what are the functions of the people from the various departments?

4.   Prioritize the actions of the physicians and nurses in the trauma situation.

B.W. is to have a CT scan of the abdomen. His abdomen has become distended and rigid.

5.   What are the possible reasons for the abdominal distention and rigidity?

6.   List 5 nursing diagnoses for this patient.

The CT scan shows a large liver laceration. B.W. will be taken directly to the OR for an exploratory laparotomy with repair of liver laceration, then to the ICU. When you return from transporting the patient to the OR, B.W.'s wife is in the ED very upset and frightened. The social worker has been called to another emergency.

7.   How would you interact with B.W.'s wife?

BIBLIOGRAPHY

Ackerman, L. (1992). Interventions related to neurologic care. *Nursing Clinics of North America, 27*(2), 325-346.

Acute Pain Management Guidline Panel. (1992). *Acute pain management: Operative or medical procedures & trauma. Clinical Practice Guideline*. Rockwell, MD: Agency for Health Care Policy & Research, Public Health Service, U. S. Department of Health and Human Services (AHCPR Pub. No. 92-0032).

American Diabetes Association. (1994). Nutrition recommendations and principles for people with diabetes mellitus (Position Statement). *Diabetes Care, 17*, 519-22.

American Heart Association. (1993). *Human blood pressure determination by sphygmometry*. Dallas, TX: Author.

American Thoracic Society/Center for Disease Control. (1990). Diagnostic standards and classification of tuberculosis. *American Review of Respiratory Disease, 142*, 725-735.

American Thoracic Society/Center for Disease Control. (1994). Treatment of tuberculosis and tuberculosis infections in adults and children. *American Journal of Respiratory Critical Care Medicine: 149,* 1359-1374.

Bachman, D. (1992). The diagnosis and management of common neurologic sequelae of closed head injury. *Journal of Head Trauma Rehabilitation, 7*(2), 50-59.

Baldwin, K., Seftchick, C., Martin, R., Sheriff, S., & Hanssen, G. (1995). *Davis's manual of critical care therapeutics*. Philadelphia: Davis.

Bartlett, J. (1995-1996). *Pocketbook of infectious disease therapy.* Baltimore: Williams & Wilkins.

Bates, B. (1991). *A pocket guide to physical examination and history taking.* Philadelphia: J. B. Lippincott.

Barton Burke, M., Wilkes, G., Berg, D., Bean, C., & Ingwersen, K. (1991). *Cancer chemotherapy: A nursing process approach.* Boston: Jones & Bartlett.

Beare, P. G., & Myers, J. L. (1994). *Adult health nursing.* St. Louis: Mosby.

Berkow, R. (Ed.). (1992). *The Merck manual of diagnosis and therapy* (16th ed.). Rahway, NJ: Merck.

Berne, R., & Levy, M. (1992). *Cardiovascular physiology* (6th Ed.). St. Louis: Mosby.

Brown, W. V. (1994). Lipoprotein disorders in diabetes mellitus. *Medical Clinics of North America, 78*, 143-161.

Brooks, S., Gochfeld, M., Herzstein, J., Schenker, M., & Jackson, R. (1995). *Environmental medicine.* St. Louis: Mosby.

Bryant, R. A. (Ed.), (1992) *Acute and chronic wounds, nursing management.* St. Louis: Mosby.

Burden, N. (1993). *Ambulatory surgical nursing.* Philadelphia: Saunders.

Burrell, L. O. (1992). *Adult nursing in hospital and community setting.* Norwalk, CT: Appleton & Lange.

Carlson, K. J., Eisenstat, S. A., Frigoletto, F. D., & Schiff, I. (Eds). (1995). *Primary care of women.* St. Louis: Mosby.

Carpenito, L. J. (1995). *Nursing diagnosis: Application to clinical practice* (6th ed.). Philadelphia: Lippincott.

Clark, J., & McGee, R. (1993). *Core curiculum for oncology nursing* (2nd ed.). Philadelphia: Saunders.

Clark, J. B. F., Queener, S. F., & Karb, V. B. (1993). *Pharmacologic basis of nursing practice.* St. Louis: Mosby.

Copstead, L. (1995). *Perspectives on pathophysiology.* Philadelphia: Saunders.

Cubbin, J. (1992). Managing resources in the community. *Nursing Standard, 7*(10), 31-34.

Cuzzell, J. Z. (1993) The right way to culture a wound. *AJN, 93*(5) 48-50.

Deglin, J., & Vallerand, A. (1993). *Davis's drug guide for nurses* (4th ed.). Philadelphia: Davis.

Devinsky, O. (1994). Seizure disorders. *Clinical Symposia, 46*(1), 2-34.

Devita, V., Hellman, S., & Rosenberg, S. (1993). *Cancer: Principles and practice of oncology* (4th ed.). Philadelphia: Lippincott.

Dodd, M. (1991). *Managing the side effects of chemotherapy and radiation.* New York: Prentice Hall.

Doughty, D., & Jackson, D. (1993) *Gastrointestinal disorders.* St. Louis: Mosby.

Driscoll, C., Bope, E., Smith, C., & Carter, B. (1996). *The family practice desk reference.* St. Louis: Mosby.

Expert Panel Report (1991). *Executive summary: Guidelines for the diagnosis and management of asthma.* National Heart, Lung, and Blood Institute, National Institutes of Health. U. S. Department of Health and Human Services. Bethesda, MD: U. S. Government Printing Services.

Fischbach, F. (1995) *Quick reference to common laboratory and diagnostic tests.* Philadelphia: Lippincott.

Folden, S. (1994). Managing the effects of a stroke: The first months. *Rehabilitation Nursing Research, 3*(3), 79-85.

Frederick, C., & Hotter, A. (1991). Discharge planning for the head-injured patient. *Critical Care Nurse, 11*(6), 42-45.

Goldberg, L., & Elliot, D. (1994). *Exercise for prevention and treatment of illness.* Philadelphia: Davis.

Groenwald, S., Frogge, M., Goodman, M., & Yarbro, C. (1993). *Cancer nursing: Principles and practice* (3rd ed.). Boston: Jones & Bartlett.

Haire-Joshu, D. (1992). *Management of diabetes mellitus: Perspectives of care across the life span.* St. Louis: Mosby.

Halstead, L. S., & Grimby, G. (1995). *Post-polio syndrome.* Philadelphia: Hanley & Belfus, Inc.

Hollander, P., Castle, G., Joynes, J. O., & Nelson, J. (1990). *Intensified insulin management for you: A personal program for advanced diabetes self-care.* Minneapolis, MN: Chronimed Publishing. [The authors are part of the International Diabetes Center in Minneapolis, MN, one of the centers involved in the Diabetes Complications and Control Trial.]

Holloway, B. (1996). *Stat facts: The clinical pocket reference for nurses.* Philadelphia: Davis.

Hudak, C., & Gallo, B. (1994). *Critical care nursing: A holistic approach.* Philadelphia: Lippincott.

International Diabetes Center. (1994). *Nutrition and diabetes: Implementing the 1994 American Diabetes Association nutrition recommendations.* Minnesota: International Diabetes Center.

Jardins, T., & Burton, G. (1995). *Clinical manifestations and assessment of respiratory disease.* St. Louis: Mosby.

Kim, M., McFarland, G., & McLane, A. (1995). *Pocket guide to nursing diagnoses* (6th ed.). St. Louis: Mosby.

Kinney, M., & Packa, D. (1996). *Andreoli's comprehensive cardiac care* (8th ed.). St. Louis: Mosby.

Kersten, L. (1989). *Comprehensive respiratory nursing.* Philadelphia: Saunders.

Lanros, N. E. (1988). *Assessment and intervention in emergency nursing.* Norwalk, CT: Appleton & Lange.

Lewis, J. (1994). *A pharmacologic approach to gastrointestinal disorders.* Baltimore, MD: Williams & Wilkins.

Lewis, S. M., & Collier, I. C. (1992). Renal and urological problems. In S. M. Lewis & I. C. Collier (Eds.), *Medical-surgical nursing: Assessment and management of clinical problems* (4th ed.). St. Louis: Mosby.

Lipman, M. M. (1993, June). Kidney stones: Painfully common, but preventable. *Consumer Report on Health,* 67.

Marrelli, T. (1994). *Handbook of home health standards and documentation guidelines for reimbursement* (2nd ed). St. Louis: Mosby.

McCance, K. L., & Huether, S. E. (1994). *Pathophysiology: The biological basis for disease in adults and children.* St. Louis: Mosby.

McCloskey, J. C., & Bulechek, G. M. (Eds.). (1992). *Iowa intervention project: Nursing interventions classification (NIC).* St. Louis: Mosby.

Metheny, N., Reed, L., Wiersema, L., McSweeney, M., Wehrle, M., & Clark, J. (1993). Effectiveness of pH measurements in predicting feeding tube placement: An update. *Nursing Research, 42*(6), 324-331.

Miller, C., & Hens, M. (1993). Multiple sclerosis: A literature review. *Journal of Neuroscience Nursing, 25*(3), 174-179.

Murphy, G., Lawrence, W., & Lenhard, R. (1995). *American Cancer Society textbook of clinical oncology* (2nd ed.). Georgia: The American Cancer Society.

National Asthma Education Program: Expert Panel Report. (1991). *Executive summary: Guidelines for the diagnosis and management of asthma.* National Heart, Lung, and Blood Institute (Publ. No. 91-3042A). Bethesda, MD: U. S. Government Printing Services.

National Cholesterol Education Program. (1993). *Second report of the National Cholesterol Education Program on detection, evaluation and treatment of high blood cholesterol in adults (adult treatment panel II).* National Heart, Lung, Blood Institute (USDHHS Publ. No. 93-3095). Bethesda, MD: U. S. Government Printing Services.

Neufeld, R. (1993). Human determination: A cherished ally in rehabilitation. *Rehabilitation Nursing, 18*(5), 326-237.

Office of Disease Prevention and Health Promotion, NIH, DHHS. (1994). *Clinician's handbook of preventive services.* Bethesda, MD: U. S. Government Printing Services.

Otto, S. (1994). *Oncology nursing* (2nd ed.). St. Louis: Mosby.

Pagana, K., & Pagana, T. (1995). *Mosby's diagnostic and laboratory test infobase.* St. Louis: Mosby.

Paul, R. (1993). *Paper prepared for the National Council for Excellence in Critical Thinking.* Rohnert Park, CA: Sonoma State University.

Phipps, W., Cassmeyer, V., Sands, J., & Lehman, M. (1995). *Medical surgical nursing-concepts and clinical practice* (5th ed.). St. Louis: Mosby

Physician's drug handbook (6th ed.) (1995). Springhouse, PA: Springhouse.

Price, S. A., & Wilson, M. W., (1992). *Pathophysiology: Clinical concepts of disease processes.* St. Louis: Mosby.

Report of the U. S. Preventive Services Task Force. (1989). *Guide to clinical preventive services: An assessment of the effectiveness of 169 interventions.* Baltimore: William & Wilkins.

Rubenstein, E., & Federman, D. (1995). *Scientific American medicine.* New York: Scientific American, Inc.

Schroeder, S., Tierney, L., McPhee, S., Papadakis, M., & Krupp, M., (1992). *Current medical diagnosis and treatment.* Norwalk, CT: Appleton & Lange

Shannon, M. T., & Wilson, B. A. (1992). *Drugs and nursing implications.* Norwalk, CT: Appleton & Lange.

Sheehy, S., & Jimmerson, C. (1994). *Manual of clinical trauma care.* St. Louis: Mosby.

Siconolfi, L. (1995) Clarifying the complexity of liver function tests. *Nursing 95, 25*(5), 39-43.

Skidmore-Roth, L. (1995). *Mosby's nursing drug infobase.* St. Louis: Mosby.

Sloane, E. (1993). *Biology of women* (3rd ed.). Department of Biological Sciences, University of Wisconsin. Milwaukee: Delmar.

Stein, J. (1994). *Internal Medicine* (4th ed.). St. Louis: Mosby.

Su, S. A. (1992). Nursing management of the larynx and tracheobronchial tree. In L. O. Burrell (Ed), *Adult nursing in hospital and community settings* (p. 755). Norwalk, CT: Appleton & Lange.

Thelan, L. A., Davie, J. K., Urden, L. D., & Lough, M. E. (1994). *Critical care nursing: Diagnosis and management.* St. Louis: Mosby.

Thompson, J. M., McFarland, G. K., Hirsh, J. E., & Tucker, S.M . (1993) Nosocomial infections. In *Mosby's clinical nursing series* (3rd ed.). St. Louis: Mosby.

Urban, N. A., Greenlee, K. K., Krumberger, J. M., & Winkelman, C. (1995). *Guidelines for critical care nursing.* St. Louis: Mosby.

Vogt, G., Miller, M., & Esluer, M. (1985). Mosby's manual of neurological care. St. Louis: Mosby.

Wachtel, T., & Stein, M. (1995). *Practical guide to the care of the ambulatory patient.* St. Louis: Mosby.

Wilson, B., Shannon, M., & Stang, C. (1995). *Nurses drug guide.* Norwalk, CT: Appleton & Lange.

Wright, J., & Shelton, B. (1993).*Desk reference for critical care nursing.* Boston: Jones & Bartlett.

Wyngaarden, J., Smith, L., & Bennett, J. (1992). *Cecil textbook of medicine* (19th ed., vol. I & II). Philadelphia: Saunders.

Zollo, A. (1995). *The portable internist.* St. Louis: Mosby.

CASE STUDY PREPSHEET

Name: _____ Date: _____ Case: _____

Symbols/terms abbreviations	Meaning/definition
_____	_____
_____	_____
_____	_____
_____	_____
_____	_____
_____	_____
_____	_____
_____	_____
_____	_____
_____	_____
_____	_____
_____	_____
_____	_____

Diagnoses (+current and -past)	Description of diagnosis
_____	_____
_____	_____
_____	_____
_____	_____
_____	_____
_____	_____

Laboratory tests and diagnostic procedures	What is it and why is it done?
_____	_____
_____	_____
_____	_____
_____	_____
_____	_____
_____	_____
_____	_____
_____	_____
_____	_____
_____	_____

439

Drugs

Generic name, class, indications, contraindications, significant side effects, food and drug interactions

_____ _____

_____ _____

_____ _____

_____ _____

_____ _____

_____ _____

_____ _____

_____ _____

_____ _____

_____ _____

_____ _____

_____ _____

_____ _____

_____ _____

_____ _____

_____ _____

_____ _____

_____ _____

_____ _____

Notes, observations, comments.

_____

_____

_____

_____

_____

_____

_____

_____

_____

_____

_____

_____

_____

_____

_____

From: Winningham, M. L., & Preusser, B. A. (1995). *Critical thinking in medical-surgical settings: A case study approach.* St. Louis: Mosby. This form may be copied if used in conjunction with this book.